PETER BENNETT

Your Spinal Health

How To Rebuild and Protect Your Central Communication System to Rebuild Your Health and Reduce Back Pain

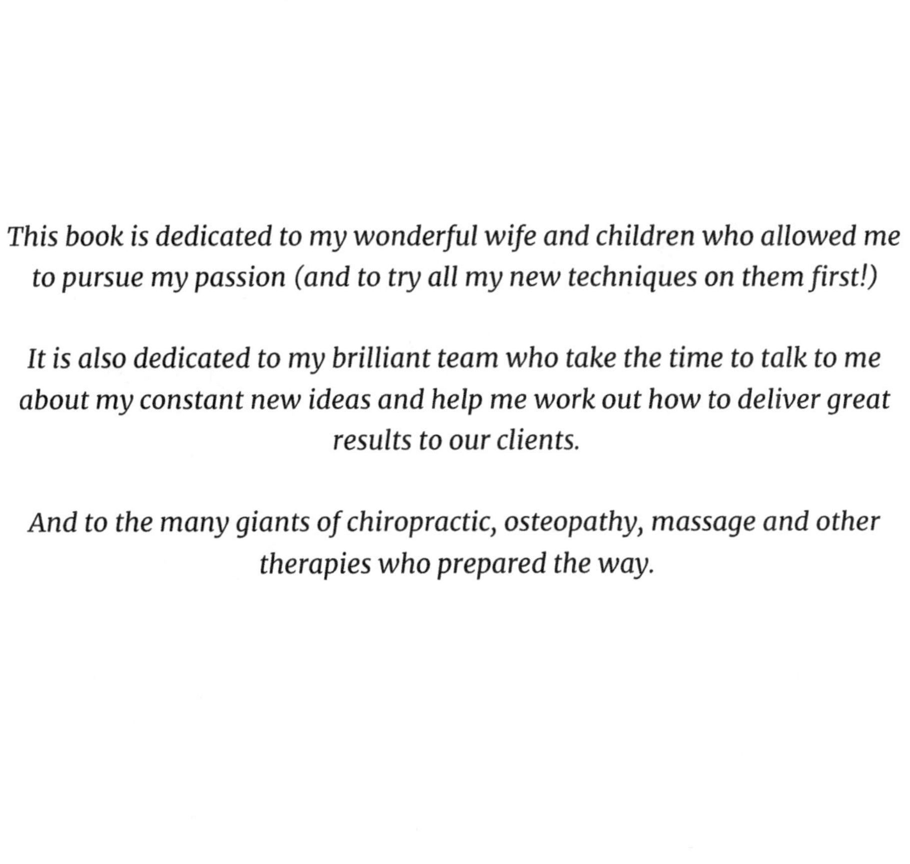

This book is dedicated to my wonderful wife and children who allowed me to pursue my passion (and to try all my new techniques on them first!)

It is also dedicated to my brilliant team who take the time to talk to me about my constant new ideas and help me work out how to deliver great results to our clients.

And to the many giants of chiropractic, osteopathy, massage and other therapies who prepared the way.

Contents

Foreword

Peter Bennett first graduated as a scientist and worked in research in academia and the pharmaceutical industry. He became a chiropractic client and was so impressed by the effect of chiropractic on his health that he enrolled in the McTimoney College of Chiropractic in Oxford, graduating in 1998.

After working in Oxfordshire he moved his family to Cumbria, where he set up Your Spinal Health in Penrith.

He and his wife and seven children all receive regular care. His children have been adjusted since birth to make sure they have an unfair advantage in life.

Preface

I started my journey in spinal health care as a chiropractic client. In my late twenties I was getting more and more painful jaw problems. Eventually I went to my GP (again) to ask her advice. She said I could either wait until I needed a jaw replacement (made me think of Jaws in the Bond movies!) or I could try a chiropractor. I had never heard the word before but I looked one up in the Yellow Pages and made an appointment.

What amazed me was that as well as sorting out my jaw my chiropractor sorted out many other health issues even though I hadn't told her about them! For example I had been getting three headaches a week from my teens. I thought this was normal so hadn't mentioned it. Although I was considered "healthy" I was getting the headaches, and the jaw pain, and the migraines, and the wobbly spells if I missed a meal, all coming from problems with the nerves in my neck. Once they were working properly my body sorted itself out.

I was so impressed I signed up to train as a chiropractor and graduated in 1998

I have been an enthusiast for chiropractic ever since. A lot of this book is about chiropractic as I know most about it. However over the years I have come to understand that there is overlap between all the various ways to work on the body and that standard chiropractic is not the only way to improve your spinal health. I have also learnt that people come to me for my help and they don't care what name I give the therapy I use.

I have learnt useful approaches from the many massage techniques, from osteopathy and physiotherapy, from sports rehabilitation and many other manual therapies. I have also learnt "mind techniques" such as life coaching and neuro linguistic programming.

What distinguishes effective therapies from ineffective therapies is the way the therapist thinks about health and about the workings of the human body.

An effective therapist takes a holistic approach. That is – everything in the body is connected to everything else, and it is all affected by the environment and by the mindset of the client. An effective therapist takes it all into account.

To this end I now work with therapists who are trained in any body work technique and show them how to think correctly about the body and how to use very specific assessment and adjustment techniques to get very effective results – which is what you as a client are really interested in. I have called this approach the Neuro Spinal Reflex Technique.

I hope that this book will give you an accurate picture of what spinal health care is, and what it isn't, and what to expect if you decide to come and see us. I also hope that it will help you if you decide not to use us.

Knowledge is power, and I am a passionate believer that your health is your greatest gift. You must have the knowledge to make your own informed decisions about how to look after your health.

If you have further questions or comments after reading this please don't hesitate to contact me.

I hope you enjoy reading this book.

Yours in health

Peter Bennett
   Chiropractor

Copyrights © Peter Bennett BSc DC

I

About Your Spinal Health

*"You are the age of your spine. You are as flexible as your spine.
That transfers to other areas of your life."*

Diane Lane

1

Why is Your Spinal Health Important?

As we move through the early years of the new century, the pace of life is becoming ever more frantic. With every passing day, there seems to be more to do than ever before. At the same time, there is little doubt that the pressure of modern life is likely to keep on increasing rather than reducing.

Because life is becoming ever more frantic and stressful, the stresses and strains on your body are also increasing on a daily basis. Your ability to deal these stresses and maintain your health is becoming more and more important.

It is little surprise that so many people are plagued with constant niggles, aches and pains. Because in our western society we most often use the medical approach of suppressing symptoms most people will take pills for their symptoms. These can cause side effects or affect health, so people take more pills to suppress the side effects of the first pills, and so on.

We are now in the strange situation where we are living longer but our health is worse, so that rather than living life to the full we live a strange sort of medicated life.

The spine is one of the major organs of the body. It is responsible for coordinating all of the other organs of the body and all the muscles, for keeping as healthy as possible and for adapting as well as possible to all the stresses and strains on the body.

Yet, if we think about it at all, we tend to think of it as merely a mechanical collection of bones. (Maybe if it was squishy like the brain or liver we would take more care of it)

Problems in the spine and nervous system take many years to show themselves as symptoms because the body works hard to adapt to injuries so we can keep going.

Some Signs of Spinal Health Problems

When symptoms do show up they can show up in a confusing variety of ways including:-
  · back pain
  · neck pain
  · headaches
  · migraines
  · sinus problems
  · immune system problems
  · balance/dizziness/vertigo
  · brain fog/concentration issues
  · low mood

All of the above can also be caused by problems with the organs. A big part of what we do as spinal therapists is to identify what are spine related problems which we can deal with, and what are organ problems which a medical doctor has to deal with.

To further confuse the issue it is perfectly possible to suffer from two or more unrelated issues at the same time. For example a person could have cancer being treated by a doctor and a spine problem being treated by a spinal therapist and a tooth problem being treated by a dentist.

Back pain is one of the more obvious spine related symptoms and it is also one of the most common reasons for people visiting their doctor.

Indeed, it has been estimated that as many as four out of every five people in the world will have to consult a medical professional at some point in their lives with a back pain problem. As only a small number of those need surgery and the medical profession can only offer medication to the rest these statistics indicate that four out of five of the population need to see a spinal therapist to solve the back problem, and the remaining one out of five should see a spinal therapist to prevent a back problem!

How Your Spinal Health Affects Your Brain Health

Your spine and your brain work together and affect each other. As we will see later your emotions will affect your spine – but your spine also affects your brain.

Your brain is constantly adapting to the signals coming to it from your body via your spine. Parts of the brain that are getting reduced signals get weaker. For example having a broken leg reduces the signal to the part of the brain that controls that leg and it grows weaker. Luckily both the leg and the brain recover quickly, but if you had reduced movement for years caused by spinal health problems the brain deterioration is longer lasting and more severe.

This may be why older people who have had reduced movement are more likely to fall - lack of feedback from the body can reduce the parts of the brain responsible for balance, coordination, reflexes and muscle strength.

This may also be why studies have shown that activities involving complex movement and coordination (such as dancing) reduce the risk of dementia and Alzheimers.

2

What Does Your Spine Do?

Your spine protects your spinal cord and nervous system and your nervous system is responsible for controlling all the systems in your body including the feedback system in your body known as "homeostasis"

Homeostasis is the process in all living things which enables them to stay healthy. All the processes in the body must be within certain limits for you to be healthy. For example if your blood got too acidic you would die. If your temperature rose too far you would die.

Your body controls everything using negative feedback loops from the body to the brain and back again. For example, in the following diagram, as soon as the temperature goes above 37 degrees sensors in your body send messages to your brain, your brain sends messages to sweat glands, you sweat and you start to cool down. Similarly if you get too cold the sensors tell your brain and the brain tells the muscles to generate heat by shivering. The same happens with your blood sugar, thyroid, blood pressure, breathing, heart rate and everything else. If you have an injury the same mechanism tells the body what to mend and when to stop.

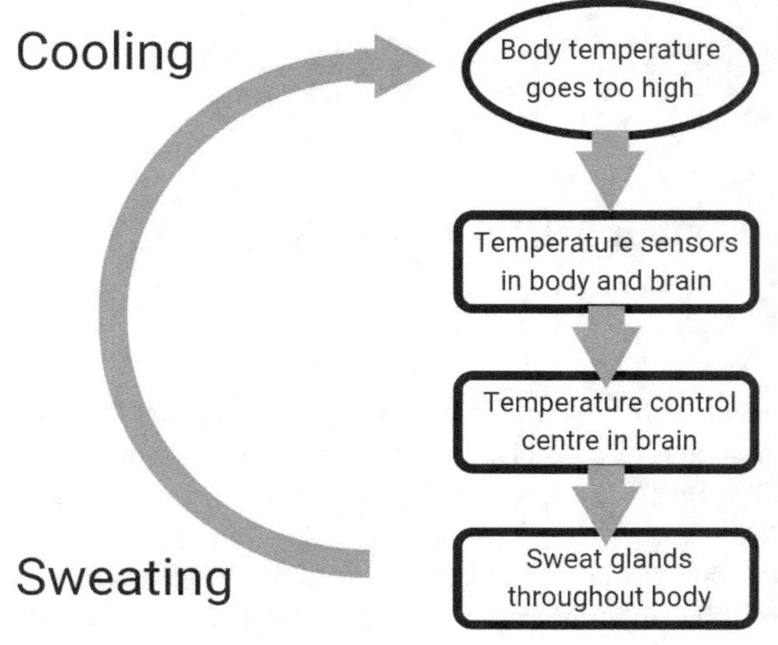

So, far from being random, our internal world is very orderly and predictable. Each living creature has an inbuilt knowledge of what it must do to survive and thrive. The circumstances in which it lives might make this impossible to do perfectly, but the knowledge is there.

Take, for example, our own bodies. When we're born we don't have learned knowledge of how to breathe, make our hearts beat, digest our food, or put everything into the right place so we can grow. Luckily our bodies know how to do all these things and the millions of other things which we have to do every second to be alive. Even as we get older, our bodies use their own innate intelligence to function as well as the situation will allow.

When you cut your finger you don't intellectually know how to make a blood clot or how to send extra white blood cells to the area to automatically fight infection. You wouldn't be able to command your body to form a scab to protect the cut area, or to grow new skin cells over the damage. But your body knows how to do these things

Your body also knows how to adapt when you're exposed to germs and viruses, eat a spoiled piece of food or strained your back lifting a heavy object. Whether it will be able to react the way it should depends on the state of your physical body

Because of genetic and environmental factors, the bodies we are born with are not always in perfect condition. In addition, the way we treat our bodies, our diet, lifestyle and emotional and mental attitudes have tremendous effects on our physical condition. If the body is limited by either inherent or acquired weaknesses innate intelligence alone will not be able to achieve perfect health. But it will always keep trying and working in that direction.

Perhaps the most important issue which can prevent proper homeostasis is spinal nerve interference, and this is where spinal health care comes in.

The body's nervous system is an incredibly complex communication network which links the brain to all parts of the body, chemically influencing even the smallest cells. There are miles of nerve fibres running throughout our bodies. No one has been able to count the number of nerve cells in the human body but it is estimated that there are at least 10 trillion to 12 trillion of them, possibly many, many more.

Over this nerve network the brain receives constantly updated information from the cells, organs and tissues and instantaneously relays instructions back. The whole process is so fast that scientists have only recently begun to measure the speed of impulses and no one has come up with a definitive speed. But you can get an idea of the incredible speed by remembering what happened last time you grabbed hold of the handle of a hot pot on the stove

Before you even realised what had happened, you jerked your hand away – and immediately a blister started forming as a protective response to the injury. You hardly had a chance to cry out in pain, but the cells in your finger had already transmitted the information about the injury to your brain which responded by instructing the cells to react in a specific way determined by your innate intelligence.

That's exactly what happens with every other cell in your body, all the time. You don't have to burn yourself to trigger the communication system. The flow of information to and from your body is a constant background function which keeps your body as healthy as it can be given its specific physical limitations.

But what if something interferes with the communication system? What if there is "line noise" as they call it in telephone circuits? What if the messages to and from the brain become even the slightest bit garbled?

The results can range from a slightly less than perfect response of a particular tissue cell, to a steadily worsening malfunction of a vital organ or life-support system. Either way, your body is not going to be able to do what its innate intelligence knows it has to do to keep up optimal health.

Below is a very simplified diagram showing the relationship between the spine, the nerves and the organs in your body.

What the nerves control

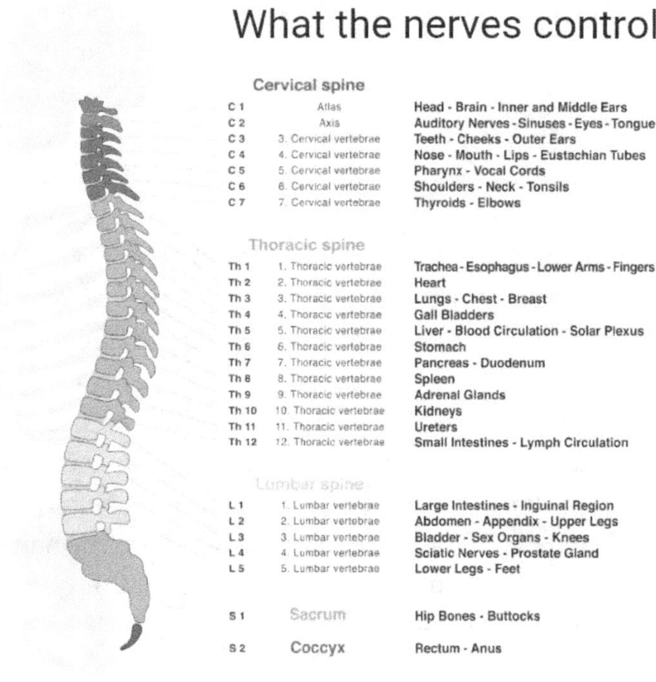

The spine is made up of 24 small bones called vertebrae: seven in the neck (cervical); 12 in the mid-back (thoracic) and five in the lower back (lumbar). Most of these vertebrae are shaped somewhat like doughnuts with a hole in the middle. The spinal cord fits into, and is protected by, these ring shaped bones. Two additional vertebrae at the bottom of the spine, the sacrum and the coccyx, complete what is called the spinal column.

Naturally nerve endings have to be able to branch out throughout the whole body, so the spinal column isn't merely a solid bone casing. Instead it is a marvel of engineering design.

The bones stack together in a precise way which allows a "canal" between them, aptly called the "neural canal". It is through this small canal that the primary nerve bundles branch off the spinal cord and make their way to all parts of the body.

If we didn't have to bend, those bones could have been locked into place. But the spine has to be flexible so its design incorporates a thick fibrous cushion of cartilage, called an intervertebral disk, which acts as a shock absorber, in the joint between each pair of vertebrae. This allows us to bend, turn, flex or move with relative freedom.

Unfortunately this need for flexibility means that the size of the canals can be made larger or smaller by movement. Think of it as a door. When the door is open all the way you can put your hand between it and the wall near the hinges. If you accidentally close the door when your hand is there, watch out! If you close it only a little bit, or quickly open it again you may escape serious injury.

But what if you don't re-open the door right away? What if you close the door on your hand and leave it closed? Before long, even if you hadn't shut the door completely - just enough to pinch your fingers - you will not only be in a great deal of pain, but you'll probably have permanently damaged your hand.

Your nerves pass through the opening in the "doorway" between the vertebrae. Usually we manage to move freely without ever closing the doorway on these nerves. But sometimes vertebrae become misaligned and the door shuts too far. Maybe not all the way, just enough to create abnormal pressure, enough to make a difference to the flow of nerve impulses through that nerve fibre. The longer the door is left partly closed the worse the damage will be.

When vertebrae become stuck in an abnormal position it's called a vertebral subluxation. To be more precise the subluxation is not merely the presence of the misaligned bone it also involves the presence of a "neurological insult" to use the technical term. In other words the misalignment is causing a change in the flow of normal impulses. The nerve "short-circuits" and is being disrupted in some way because of the misaligned bones.

The effects of vertebral subluxation on health have been well-documented in the millions of case studies recorded by practising chiropractors. It is the spinal health therapist's job to determine whether there are any subluxations and to introduce the precise amount of force, called an adjustment, to gently but firmly unlock the vertebrae and allow them to return to the proper alignment.

Of course there are other things that can interfere with proper flow of nerve impulses. Among these are chemicals, such as those found in certain food and drinks, pollutants and even prescription and over-the-counter drugs. In fact early chiropractors were the first "body ecologists" to sound an alarm about the damage which could be done by the unwise use of chemicals dumped into the most important stream in the world - the human bloodstream.

3

Your Spinal Contour And Good Posture

Whether you are sitting, standing, working, sleeping or relaxing; your spine is most comfortable in what is called a neutral posture - properly balanced and using least energy.

In the neutral position your spine has three natural curves: the inward curve at the neck (cervical lordosis), the outward curve at the upper back (thoracic kyphosis), and finally the inward curve at the low back (lumbar lordosis).

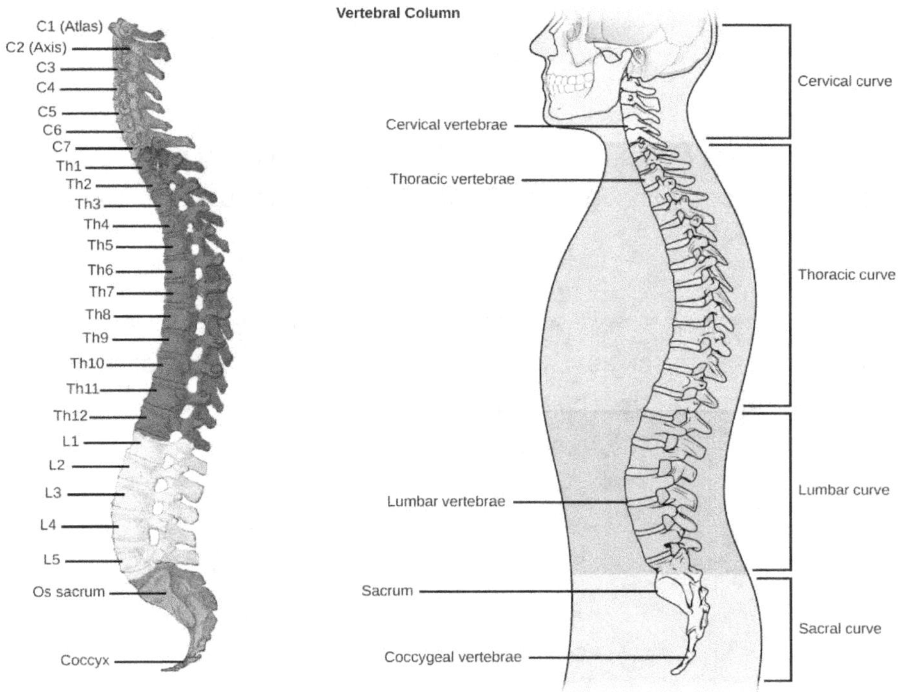

The neutral spinal curves differ in shape from person to person. Neutral spinal curves can change for the better with exercise and training; And sometimes for the worse with injury, aging, poor posture habits or a disease.

The amount of curving in your spine when you are in a neutral posture determines your support needs. A spinal support product should be deep enough to support your particular curves without pushing beyond your neutral postures. Meaning it should feel natural and not too arched; you should also feel supported; meaning there must not be a gap between you and the support.

Scoliosis

When you look at the spine from the back it should be straight. Often an early sign of spinal health problems is side to side curves in the spine known as scoliosis.

This is an X-ray of severe scoliosis. Most cases aren't as severe as this but you can see the strain this would put on the structures of the spine and how this could tire the muscles.

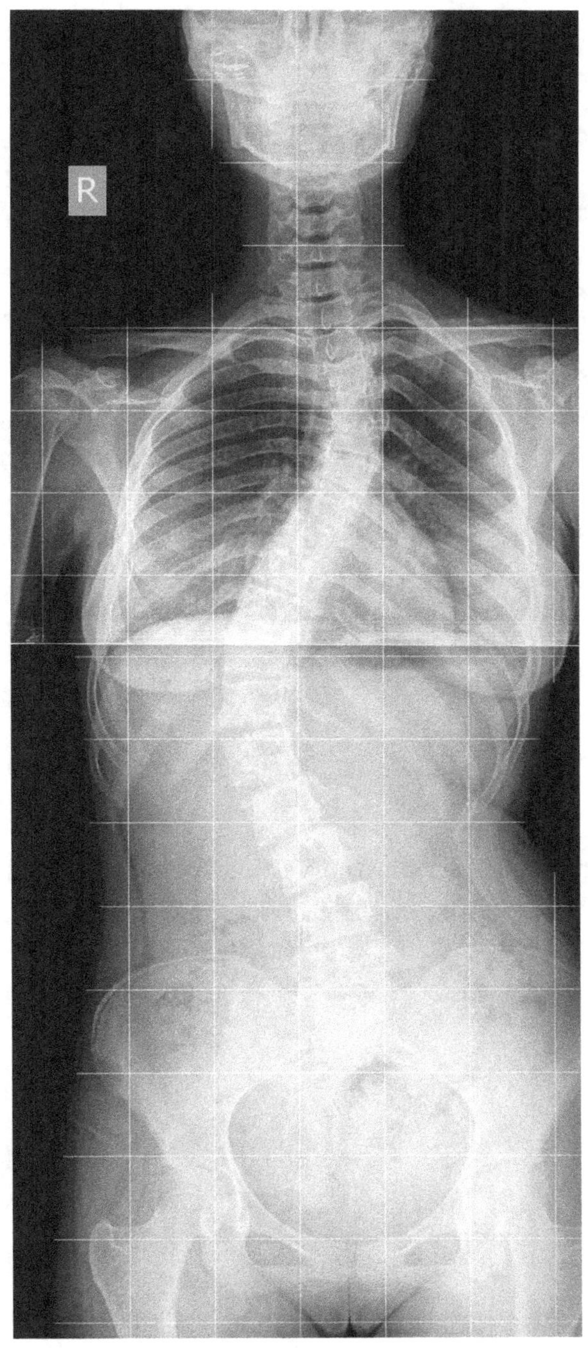

An Example of Severe Scoliosis

Symptoms of scoliosis can include:-
- Bump in the lower back
- Numbness, weakness, or pain in the legs
- Trouble walking
- Trouble standing up straight
- Tired feeling
- Shortness of breath
- Loss of height
- Bone spurs — bony bumps in the joints of the spine from bone and joint damage
- Feeling full quickly while you eat. This is because your spine is putting pressure on your belly.

Kyphosis

Excessive forward or backward curvature is called kyphosis. It is easiest to see in people who have thoracic kyphosis

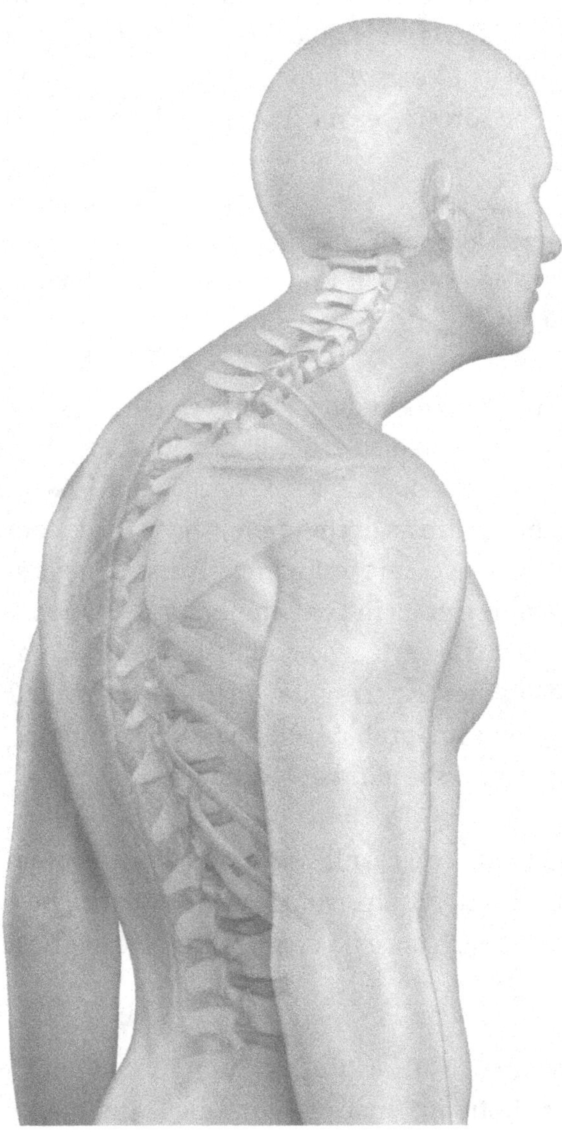

Kyphosis

Types of Kyphosis

Postural kyphosis is the most common type. In the young, it can be called "slouching" and is reversible by correcting muscular imbalances. In the old, it may be a case of hyperkyphosis and called "dowager's hump". This is the sort we see most often and it often responds well to care.

The other forms of kyphosis respond less well to spinal care. We aim to keep the spine in as good a condition as possible and to slow down deterioration if possible.

Scheuermann's kyphosis is significantly worse and can cause varying degrees of pain, and can also affect different areas of the spine (the most common being the upper back. Scheuermann's kyphosis is a form of juvenile osteochondrosis of the spine, and is more commonly called Scheuermann's disease. It is found mostly in teenagers and presents a significantly worse deformity than postural kyphosis. Whereas in postural kyphosis, the vertebrae and discs look normal, in Scheuermann's kyphosis, they are irregular and often damaged. Fatigue is a very common symptom, probably because of the intense muscle work that has to be put into standing or sitting properly.

Congenital kyphosis can result in infants whose spinal column has not developed correctly in the womb. Vertebrae may be malformed or fused together and can cause further progressive kyphosis as the child develops.

Nutritional kyphosis can result from nutritional deficiencies, especially during childhood, such as vitamin D deficiency (producing rickets), which softens bones and results in curving of the spine and limbs under the child's body weight.

Post-traumatic kyphosis can arise from untreated or ineffectively treated vertebral fractures. This can happen in older people with osteoporosis.

4

Causes of Spinal Problems

It can be difficult to trace the exact cause of spinal pain. In many cases the initial injury that set in motion the chain of events that led to the pain was many years before and in a different part of the body. For example, an unresolved knee injury can lead to distortion in the spine which eventually causes neck pain.

We need to sort out the original problem if we are to get to proper spinal health.

The root causes can be physical (old injuries), chemical (a toxin causing stress in the system for example) or mental (a long period of chronic stress for example)

All of these stresses can cause compensatory twisting in the spine, which leads to weak spots and further compensation, until your body cries "enough" and gives you pain as a warning.

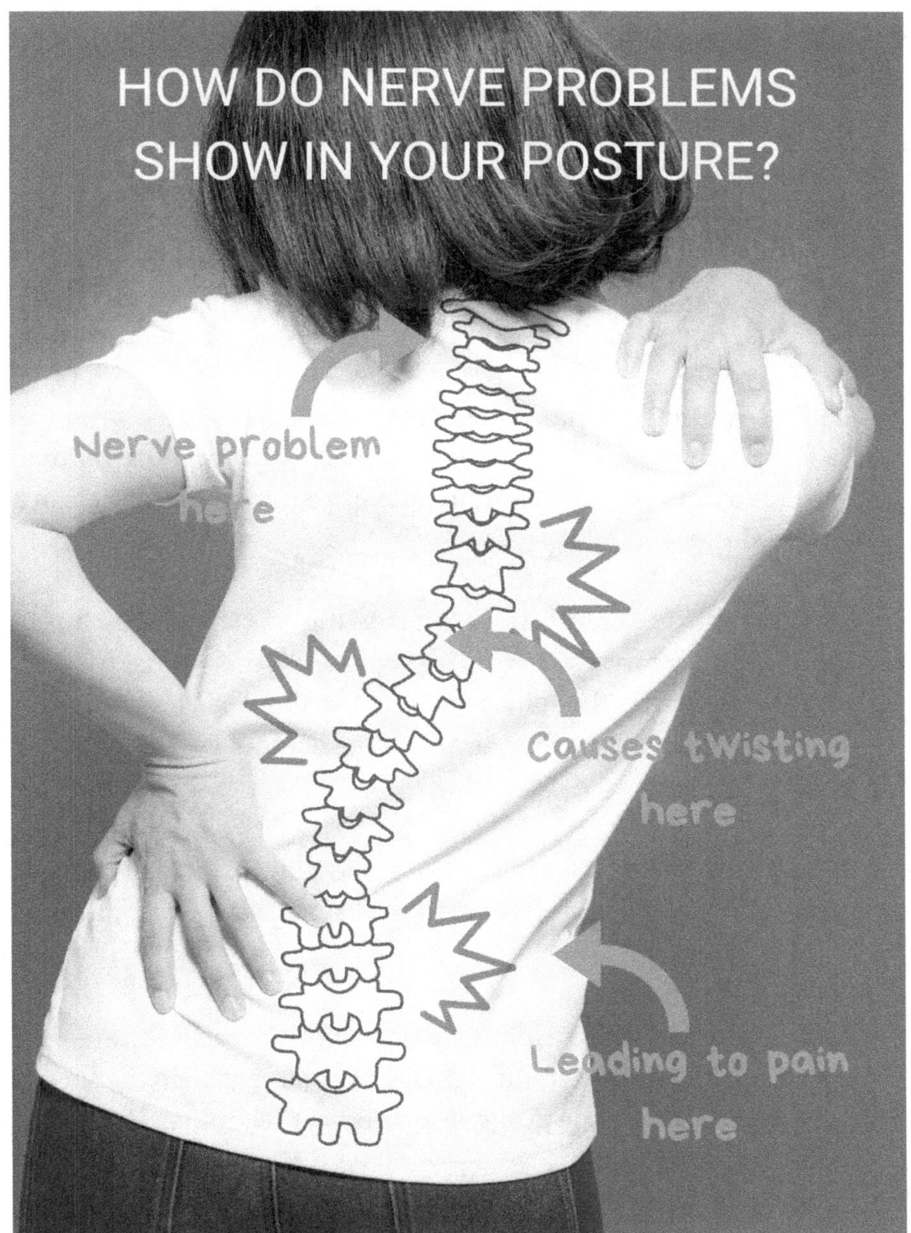

HOW DO NERVE PROBLEMS
SHOW IN YOUR POSTURE?
Nerve problem here
Causes twisting here
Leading to pain here

When pain eventually appears it is usually triggered by one of these problems:

- Muscle Spasm – Spasms around the spine can be caused by injuries or strains that trigger the body to flex or contract the muscles in order to protect the affected areas.

- Arthritis – Spinal arthritis can cause stiffness and inflammation.

- Herniated Disc(s) – The vertebral discs contain fluid that serves as padding between each vertebra. And when a disc, or discs, become herniated or ruptured, the fluid puts pressure on the spinal cord and produces pain.

- Spinal Stenosis – Stenosis or "narrowing" of the spaces in the spinal column can result from arthritis and other spinal injuries. Stenosis constricts the spinal cord and therefore causes numbness and pain throughout the lower part of the body and even up to your arms.

- Spondylolisthesis – The spinal vertebrae can slip out of place and press onto the underlying nerves, so it causes sharp pain and even numbness.

- Spinal Infection – Severe injuries to the spine can cause an infection to develop in the spinal fluids. This is a serious problem that needs to be treated or else the progression of the infection might lead to paralysis or debilitation.

- Kidney Stones – Though kidney stones don't directly affect the spine, it can cause radiating pain across the lower back, sides, and abdomen.

-

- Bone cancer and bone infections

Spinal therapists are trained in identifying what issues we can help with and which (bone infections and kidney stones for example) have to be dealt with medically.

In many cases over the years clients have come to me with a diagnosis of, for example, low back pain caused by a bulging lumbar disc. They have had years of lower back treatment which hasn't worked. As we worked together we found that the bulging disc was actually a compensation for misalignment in their neck. The previous treatments hadn't worked because they were working on where the **symptom** was rather than where the **problem** was! By taking a whole body approach and listening to the body we were able to help the real problem and get them better.

Of course there have been people we haven't been able to help but we are always careful to identify when there is a problem and send the client back to their doctor for further tests.

5

A Brief History of Your Symptoms?

As I noted in the previous chapter your spinal health doesn't usually change from perfect health to symptoms in one moment, unless you have fallen from a great height or been in a major car accident for example.

With the majority of my clients there has been a history of accidents and stresses over many years. Their spines have twisted and turned, sometimes showing symptoms and sometimes not, but eventually building up enough damage that they have severe enough symptoms that they can't stand it any more and they are looking for an answer.

Spinal degeneration has been studied for many years and there is a very typical pattern that most people follow. The spinal degeneration goes through four phases: -

DEGENERATION PHASE 1

During the first stage of spinal degeneration a minor loss of spinal curvature and normal balance may be experienced. This leads to stress of the surrounding features of the spine such as disc, joints, nerves and posture causing them to age faster. Because the body is so adaptable, this phase might present with no warning of pain or other symptoms.

With proper care, there is an excellent chance of reducing or reversing the degeneration in this phase.

DEGENERATION PHASE 2

By the second stage of spinal degeneration, you are likely to experience pain, aches, stress, and fatigue. There is a much greater degree of decay, bone spurs, disc narrowing, and postural changes are much worse due to the lack of normal joint movement. Decreased disc height and spinal canal narrowing or stenosis may occur. This condition is very common in 80% of males and 76% of females by the age of 40. It is vital that these symptoms are not ignored as care during this phase can lead to significant improvement.

DEGENERATION PHASE 3

After years of neglect you will probably experience a loss of energy, loss of height, increased nerve damage, restriction of motion, abnormal curvature of the spine, more postural imbalances, permanent scar tissue and advanced bone deformation.

The situation can still be improved with care but it can take longer and reactions are more frequent because there is more damage to heal.

DEGENERATION PHASE 4

This is the most advanced form of degeneration. The postural imbalance is severe and motion is limited. Most of the damage that as occurred in this stage is now permanent. There is severe nerve damage, massive calcium damage, permanent scar tissue has formed and bones may begin to fuse. This results from long term neglect of spinal misalignment. At this point we can offer pain management and treatments to increase your comfort levels.

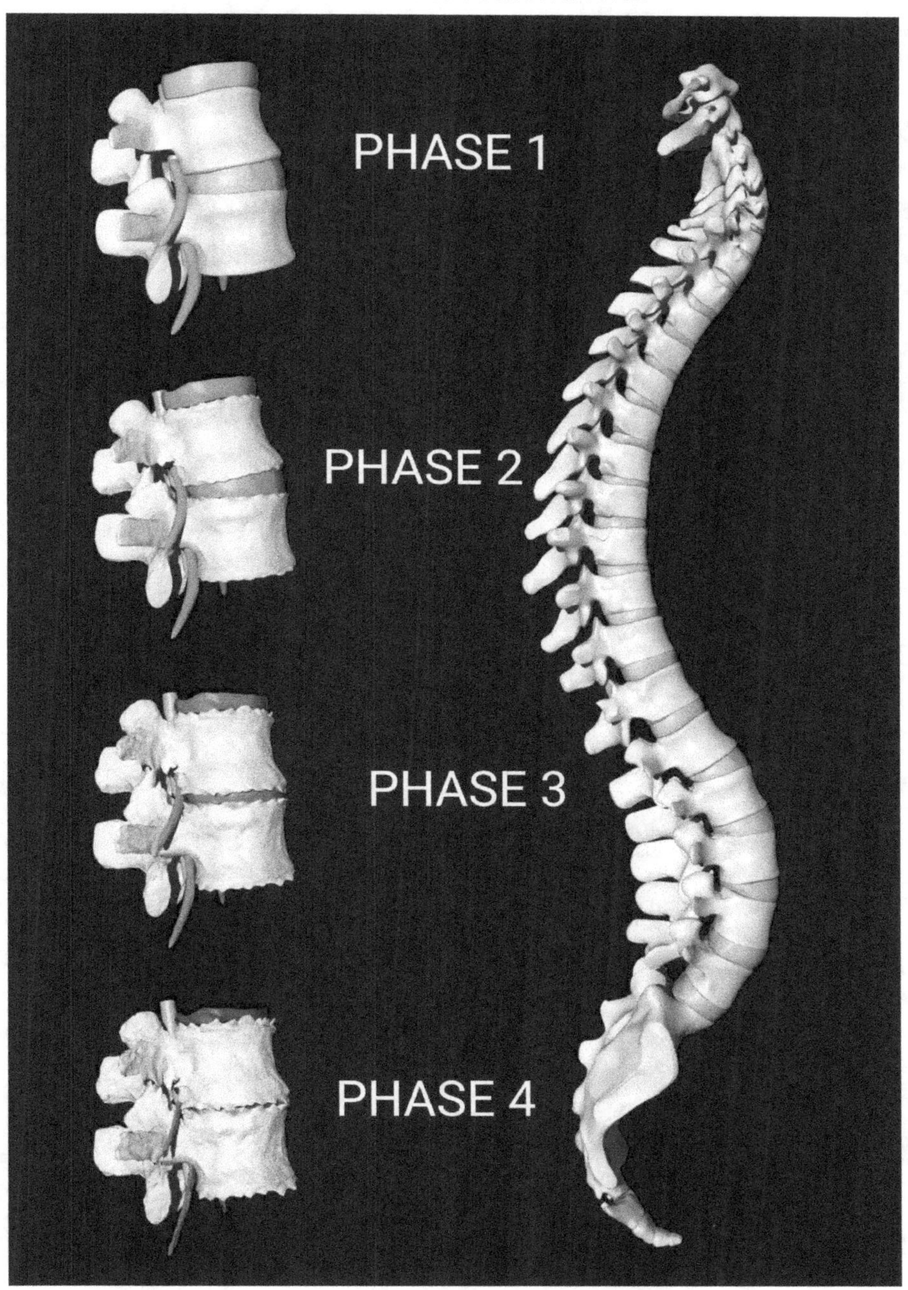

PHASE 1
PHASE 2
PHASE 3
PHASE 4

On average getting enough damage to show up on an MRI scan takes about 10 years.

Even when damage can be seen symptoms do not always show up immediately or in a obvious way. Often people will experience vague symptoms like "feeling under the weather" or " feeling out of sorts" or just tired.

Your body will always tell you if there is a problem, but sometimes it starts by whispering to you and if that doesn't work it will start screaming at you.

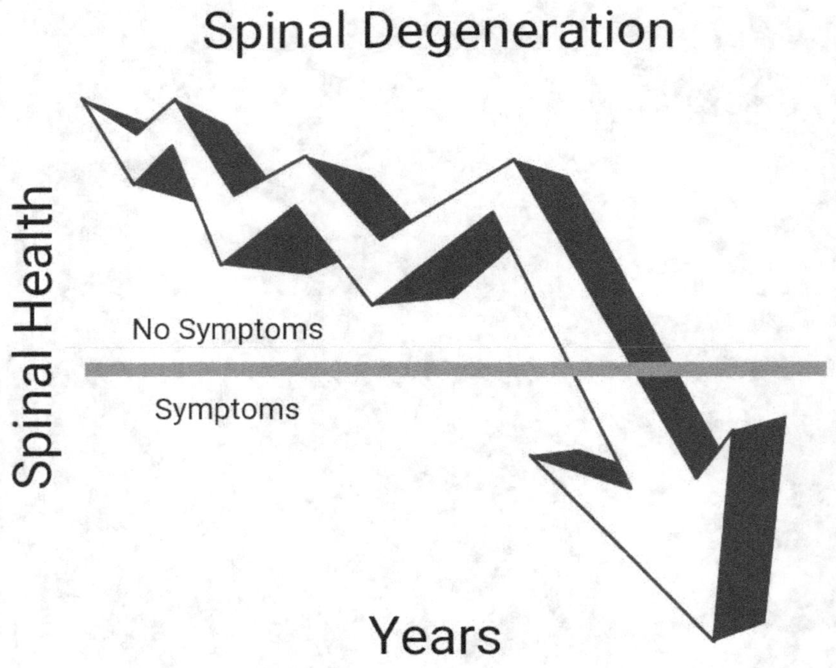

6

What Are The Benefits of Maintaining a Healthy Spine?

- You'll have more resistance to injury because your muscles, ligaments and discs are stronger.
- You'll get greater benefit from exercise because you're not wasting any energy, and your muscles and ligaments are working properly.
- Your organs will work better because they have less stress on them and the nerves to them will be working properly.
- Your nervous system will work better, which means that everything to do with your nervous system will work better. Your reflexes will be faster, you'll heal faster, and you will think better.
- The self-healing system depends on the brain being aware of where the damage is in the body. It does this through the nervous system, which goes through the spine. If your spine is stronger and straighter, your nerves will work better, and you will heal faster.
- You'll have greater flexibility, and might be able to touch your toes for the first time in a long time!
- You will have more energy because you won't be wasting any energy in excessive muscle tension, and your systems will be working at maximum efficiency.
- As well as less wear and tear on the spine, you will get less wear and tear on your hips and knees and your ankles because your pressure

distribution will be more even.

- You will get less back ache and neck ache because you will have less muscle strain and less muscle inflammation in and around the spine.
- You will get fewer headaches and migraines because you will be getting less muscle tension in your neck and improved blood flow and nerve supply into your brain.

7

Why Transforming Your Health is Difficult

Whenever you try to change a habit you will resist it. Your body has got used to the situation you have been experiencing and it has found a way of dealing with it and keeping your body as healthy as possible.

This is true even if the situation is bad for your health, drinking too much or smoking for example. If you have ever tried to change a habit you will have experienced this resistance. Your body starts craving what you want to give up and your mind starts to justify the habit "I need this because..."

You could think of this resistance as gravity. For a rocket to escape gravity and get into space it has to put a lot of energy into the first 10 minutes of take off. Once it has achieved escape velocity it can cruise the rest of the way with just little bursts of energy to alter course.

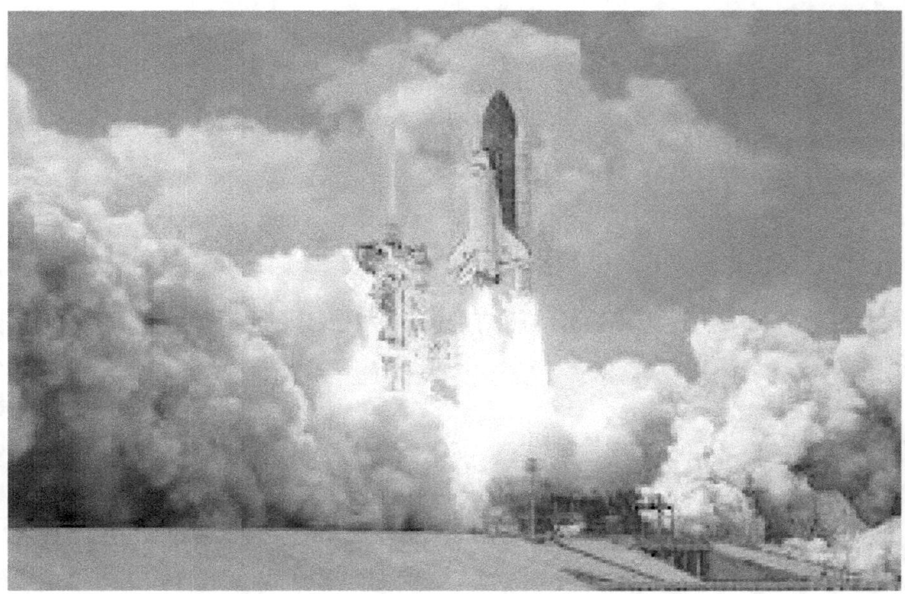

When you change a habit it is easy in the first few days because it is new and interesting. After a few days the resistance starts and it takes a great effort of willpower to keep going. If you can put in the required effort for 30 days your body starts to get used to the new situation and you don't have to put in so much effort – you have achieved escape velocity!

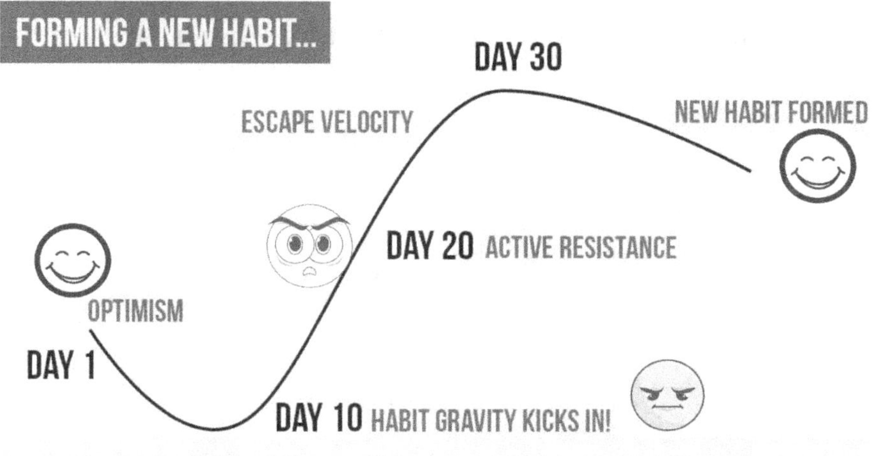

Acquiring a new habit always takes time

Over the years your spine has adapted to the stresses and strains on it by altering its' posture and growing the muscles, ligaments and discs to suit that posture. Your brain will also have got used to that posture and will think of that as normal.

When treatment starts your posture will straighten up. Your brain has to be retrained to accept the new straight posture and your muscles, ligaments and discs will have to regrow into the new positions.

This is why the whole process of getting your spinal health up to the best possible level takes 12 weeks and why you need intensive treatment over the first 30 days to get your body into the new habit of staying straight.

It also shows why new clients very often go through a discouraged phase around weeks 2 and 3. Resistance to change is built into the system and about weeks 2 and 3 it starts to kick in as your body and mind complain about having to change everything. Once you get through this phase your body starts to accept and welcome the changes and it feels easier again.

8

Improve Your Health or Reduce Your Symptoms?

We make sure that your spine and nervous system are working at their best so that everything works at maximum efficiency and you are in the best health possible. It is a simple concept.

So why do people get confused about what spinal health care is?

There are a number of reasons

First there are all those testimonials from satisfied clients. Of course we love to hear from clients who are feeling healthier and happier because of regular spinal health care care. But, as we mentioned before, some clients forget the most important important part of the story – that correcting the spine allows the intelligence that made the body to heal the body. In their enthusiasm they give credit to the spinal health therapist for their "cures".

When a client tells a friend that her child's ear infections were "cured" by spinal health care the friend is bound to get the impression that the spinal health therapist diagnosed the child's condition and specifically treated it. The same thing goes when a client tells a co-worker that his migraines disappeared after only a few adjustments. The co-worker will go home thinking spinal health care is a treatment for headaches.

When the friend and the co-worker go to see the spinal health therapist themselves, they are going to be expecting their spinal health therapist to diagnose their illnesses and treat them. When they're told that the purpose of spinal health care is to determine whether they have problems in their spine and correct them, they are bound to be confused.

One way to avoid this confusion is for us to make sure that clients have proper educational material- hence this book.

For their part clients have to play an active role in their own healthcare and take time to learn about and understand spinal health care.

This isn't easy because for decades we've been made to be spectators when it comes to health. We sit back and put our health into the hands of the experts. Studies have shown that the vast majority of clients who go to a medical doctor never ask a single question about the doctor's diagnosis or treatment plan. They never ask about the drugs they are given, not even about potential side-effects they may experience. Most are too intimidated to demand a second opinion even in the case of the diagnosis of serious illness. This is as much a problem for the medical doctor as it is the client. If there is no dialogue the doctor can miss out on important information.

Your health is too important not to ask questions about your care, your spinal health care care or your medical care. If you don't take the time to understand what they can do for you and how they are going to do it you're not going to get as much out of it as those people who are well informed, and you risk the dissatisfaction that comes with misunderstanding.

The role of a doctor is to keep you alive with surgery, pills and other "outside in" procedures. They will treat pain with painkillers, depressions with anti- depressants and so on.

The role of a spinal therapist is to keep you so healthy you don't need the symptoms. We don't diagnose disease or treat symptoms - we help your body's natural healing mechanisms.

In our practice we try to keep this as clear as possible. This is why we don't wear white coats, and we don't use stethoscopes or any medical equipment. Our clients see us for spinal health issues, and their medical doctor for medical issues.

II

A Brief History of Spinal Health Care

"Natural forces within us are the true healers of disease."

Hippocrates

9

Spine Care Through The Ages

Spinal health care treatments (although not named as such) have existed for a very long time. Many civilizations have evidence which suggest that this type of treatment was used.

A Chinese text dating back to 2700 BC suggests that such techniques were being used.

A papyrus found in Egypt dating back to 1600 BC describes a treatment for a dislocated jaw.

Various other societies including ancient Babylon, Tibet, Syria, Japan, India and even some North American tribes and South American groups have been using such treatments.

The ancient Indian practice of Yoga concentrated on keeping the spinal column flexible through various exercises, there is an old yogic saying that 'a person is only as healthy as his spine'.

Around 2400 years ago in 400 BC, Hippocrates (considered to be "the father of medicine") founded a school in ancient Greece. Hippocrates believed that ill health was a result of improper diet, surrounding environment, our lifestyle and the effect of these on the spine.

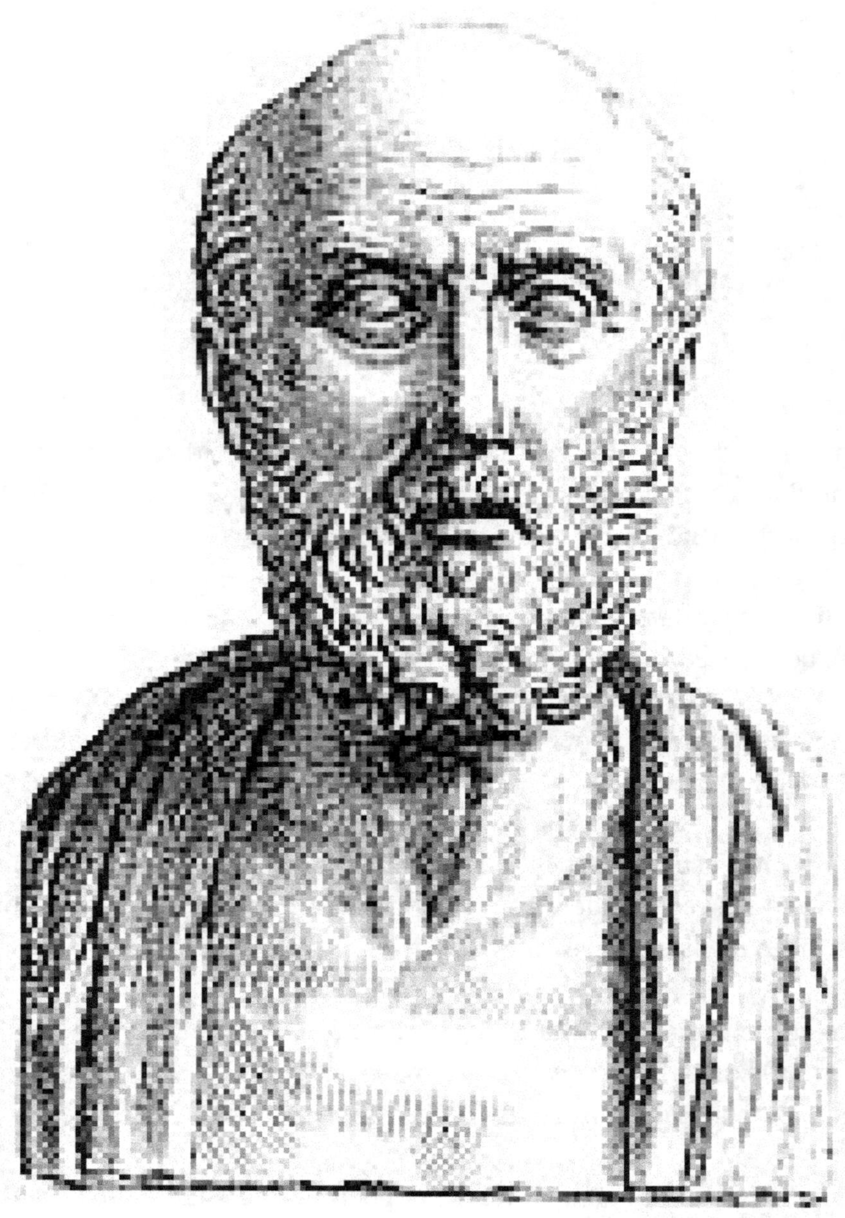

Hippocrates

Hippocrates is known for dealing with the plague that hit Athens in 430- 427 BC, and for healing the king of Macedonia's tuberculosis. He is also known for his book the Hippocrates Corpus which contains at least seventy of his best works.

Hippocrates also documented the key role of the spine and nervous system. He wrote – " Get knowledge of the spine, for this is the requisite for many diseases.' Hippocrates' many writings included manuscripts such as ' Manipulation and Importance of Good Health ' and another called ' Setting Joints By Leverage '. These works were written around 500 B.C.

Physicians who followed Hippocrates relied on nature's healing power to improve health. They focussed on diet, exercise, rest to improve the health of a client.

Another famous Greek Physician, Galen, wrote early in the second century – "Look to the nervous system as the key to maximum health". Galen was made famous for treating a Roman scholar. He adjusted Eudemus' neck which cured a paralysis of the scholar's hand and arm. Galen is also credited with the following wisdom – 'Leaving the affected parts alone, you will reach the spine from which you will treat the disease.'

One of the basic and natural methods for healing the human body according to Hippocrates was correction of the spine. Hippocrates is known to have said that "physical structure is the basis of medicine". He established a detailed study of how changes in health can occur if the structure of the spine is damaged.

Hippocrates had immense knowledge about complete and partial dislocations of bones as suggested in most of his texts. One text even mentions the procedure of reducing a client's hump by making him lie flat on a soft material applying force on his hump. This could either be done with the hand, foot or even a board.

Kingdoms of ancient Greece and Roman Empires followed Hippocratic studies and methods very closely. Since physical fitness was important in their kingdoms and half of the men were warriors by profession, it was imperative for them to look after themselves with proper diet and exercise. However, as empires fell most of the knowledge they gained from Hippocrates was lost. However, copies and texts continued to circulate with the help of monks and Islamic physicians living in faraway monasteries, seminaries and mosques around the world.

In Europe during the 1800's medical doctors shunned the art of "bone-setting" instead tending to use dramatic treatments such as purging with laxatives, bloodletting, and cupping (heated glasses placed on the affected areas to get rid of tumours), applying leeches and cauteries (hot irons) to the skin over tender spinal areas. But in 1867 a famous surgeon, Sir James Paget, recognised the evolving art with his article in the British Medical Journal entitled , 'Cases That Bone-Setting Cures'. In it he described the types of spinal manipulation known at the time. In the early part of the 20th century Germany enjoyed a thriving branch of manual medicine.

Ordinary people who didn't have access to doctors required the help of folk or lay practitioners. These practitioners included herbalists and bonesetters. Bonesetters in the past could not only fix broken bones of the arms and legs, but also had enough training to perform adjustment of the spine and other joints. They were very popular in the past in European countries for their various practices. One of the most popular bonesetters in the eighteenth century.was actually not a man, but a woman - Sally Map. In Cumbria bonesetters continued to practice very successfully up to the last 20 years.

Physiotherapy as a profession started primarily with Per Henrik Ling (known as the "Father of Swedish Gymnastics") who founded the Royal Central Institute of Gymnastics (RCIG) in 1813 for massage, manipulation, and exercise.

In the USA in the late 1800's there was a lot of interest in medicine and alternative medicine. Ancient texts from the East and from ancient Greece and Rome were more widely available for study. Louis Pasteur had published his Germ Theory in 1861 which demonstrated that many diseases are caused by microscopic organisms called pathogens (bacteria and viruses). However many people were already questioning why, if all that is needed for a disease is a pathogen, doesn't everyone exposed to the pathogen get the disease. The developers of alternative medicine at that time were looking at ways to increase the strength of the body so that it could fight the pathogen more effectively.

The first school of osteopathy was founded in 1922 by Andrew Taylor Still in Kirksville, Missouri. He started developing his ideas in the 1890's.

The first chiropractic college was Palmer College of Chiropractic, established in 1897 by Daniel David Palmer in Davenport, Iowa.

Many different approaches and techniques have been developed over the years by chiropractors, osteopaths and physiotherapists. The aim of all of these approaches is to get the best results for the client.

Many people get confused about whether they should go to a medical doctor or to a spinal therapist.

My approach is that medical approaches work best with acute, life threatening issues like heart disease, trauma (car accidents, broken bones) and organ related diseases. In other words medicine tries to bring to bring you back from the brink and keep you alive.

Spinal therapy aims to restore the spine and nervous system to full strength so that everything is working at its' best. This does not mean that you never get a disease or an accident that requires medical care, but it makes your body better at fighting disease and repairing itself.

10

What Is The Neuro Spinal Reflex Technique?

I developed the Neuro Spinal Reflex Technique over 20 years in practice as I sought constantly to improve in three areas:-
   1. To be gentler
   2. To be more effective
   3. To be more precise

NEURO SPINAL REFLEX TECHNIQUE

An advanced, highly specific, micro massage technique which corrects the spine by activating neuro spinal reflexes

The guiding principle behind this approach is that your body knows exactly what it is doing and it always does everything to be as healthy as possible. It is based to a large extent on the chiropractic approach but brings in elements from other professions and ways of thinking.

So even when there is a symptom there is always a good reason why you are having the symptom.

- If you are in pain your body is trying to stop you causing more damage
- If you are vomiting or have diarrhoea your body is trying to clear out a toxin
- If you have a temperature your body is trying to kill off a virus
- If you have a twist in your spine your body is trying to keep pressure off a nerve

Another way of looking at this is that your body has "innate intelligence". In other words it is born knowing what to do.
- It knows how to grow from one cell to where you are now
- It knows how to heal an injury
- It knows how to fight off infections
- It knows how to digest food
- It knows how to clear out toxins

Imagine what would happen if you suddenly needed outside help to carry out all the functions you now do automatically. No doctor or medical procedure would even come close to managing it.

How would you do if you had to consciously organise all the different things your body is doing second by second?

Our approach starts from a deep respect for the healing power of the body and a desire to listen to its' wisdom.

Unfortunately the medical approach often seems to have no respect for the body - treating it as a faulty machine that needs to be forced into doing the "right" thing.

The medical approach works best in life-threatening emergencies like car accidents and open heart surgery - yet would surgery work if the body didn't have the power to heal the wounds?

So how does the body know what needs to be done and where?

The body is a complex network of biofeedback loops which in simple terms can thought of as a reflex.

A simple reflex is the one your doctor will test by tapping your kneecap with a rubber hammer.

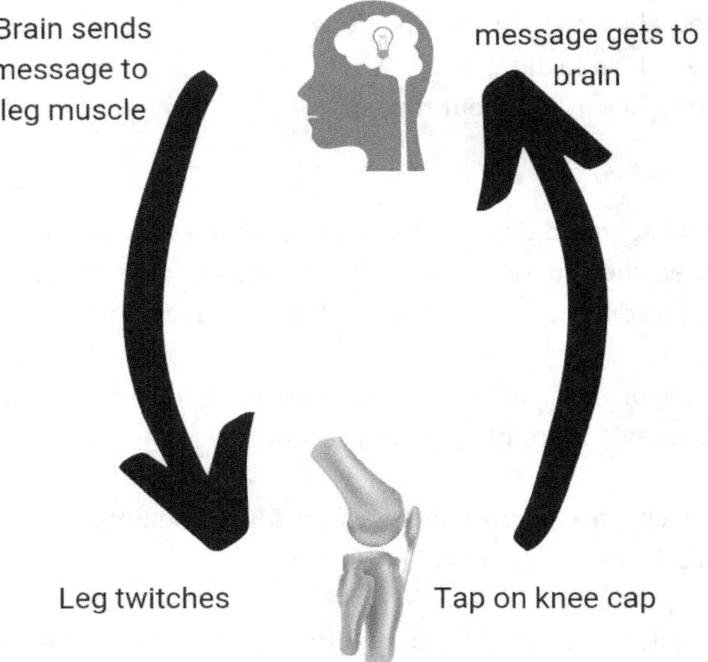

A more subtle reflex can be used to find out whether a particular point in your back needs to be adjusted.
  - If I touch that point the message goes to your brain.
  - If there is a problem at that point the brain sends a reflex and your body flinches. The change in body structure can be detected by a change in leg length for example.
  - Your body can tell me exactly what it needs in this way
  - I can then deliver a gentle stimulus in the right place
  - Your brain receives the message and decides whether it is safe to move the bone into a new position. If it isn't safe nothing happens
  - I recheck your body to see whether your body has accepted the

change or not

This process is repeated until your whole body has been checked and corrected.

People are often surprised by the speed and efficiency of the technique. Checking the whole body and nervous system usually takes between 5 and 10 minutes.

The whole process involves reflexes between the brain and nervous system (neuro) and the spine – hence Neuro Spinal Reflex Technique.

Because the technique is gentle and safe it can be taught to any therapist who has sufficient knowledge of anatomy, physiology and is suitably qualified in a body therapy.

III

How to Improve Your Spinal Health

"My body is damaged from music in two ways. I have a red irritation in my stomach. It's psychosomatic, caused by all the anger and the screaming. I have scoliosis, where the curvature of your spine is bent, and the weight of my guitar has made it worse. I'm always in pain, and that adds to the anger in our music."

Kurt Cobain

11

Putting All The Ingredients For Health Together

There are three main pillars to spinal health

Physical – which includes
- Spinal realignment (the adjustment)
- Relaxing over-tight muscles
- Strengthening weak muscles
- Exercises for muscles, tendons and ligaments

Chemical – which includes
- Eating the right foods
- Avoiding toxins
- Drinking enough water

Mental – which includes
- Stress management
- Dealing with emotional scar tissue and trauma
- Dealing with mental habits

There is a huge amount of information around about all of these issues.

However usually everything is dealt with in isolation – diet books don't tend to address emotional issues for example.

Imagine getting to better health was a wall you had to climb up. You can collect three blocks called physical, chemical and mental, but if you don't stack them together properly they don't help you climb the wall.

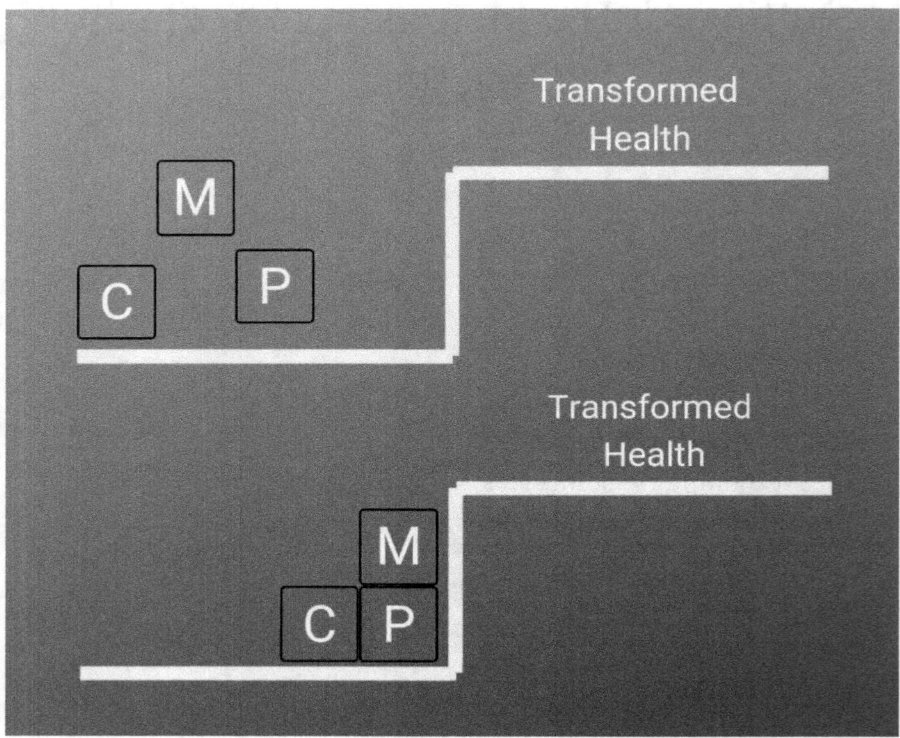

This is why our approach is holistic – we need to link everything together to get you to higher level health.

12

The Spinal Health Care Examination

As you have read, the focus of spinal health care is to improve your health by detecting and correcting vertebral subluxations (interference to your nerves) and problems in and around your spine.

Therefore our examinations are aimed very specifically at this focus.

The initial questionnaire is designed to get as much information as possible to help us decide whether you should come to us, or whether you should see your GP in the first instance.

The examinations are designed to find the effect of spinal problems on your body.

Physical Examination

This will include the following tests

Range of motion.

One of the effects of the subluxation is to impair voluntary movement (called dyskinesia"). In clients this usually means difficulty turning their head or body from side to side or front to back. Often clients will be able to turn to the left a lot further than they can to the right or vice versa. This impaired range of motion can be tested and measured very accurately.

Postural checks

The way you hold your body can be a good indication of the proper alignment of the spine. We will visually check various reference points and note the tilt and balance of each. A client who stands with one shoulder higher than the other, for example, might have a severe vertebral subluxation which could cause serious health damage.

Leg length check

If your body is compensating for subluxations in your spine you will twist yourself and you will end up with one leg longer than the other. Most people have one leg longer than the other, but this is because most people are subluxated. People under our care always have even leg length, (unless they have had leg surgery or a bad fracture)

Palpation

After years of training and clinical practice spinal therapists learn to "feel" for subluxations in the spine with the tips of the fingers. Most are remarkably accurate with this type of examination and can also become aware of any tenderness, soreness or discomfort experienced by the client as a result of having vertical subluxations.

We explain what we have found, and what we can do about it. You then decide whether to carry on with care.

13

Top 10 Tips for Preventing Spine Pain

LISTEN TO YOUR BACK

Pain is a warning sign. Your body is telling you that you have already or are about to cause damage. If what you are doing hurts then STOP. Do not try to push through the pain.

EXERCISE

Regular exercise is important to help maintain mobility and strength. It should be done without pain and it should be done regularly. Brisk walking, swimming and cycling are all excellent exercises, but you should do what is suitable for you and what you enjoy. See the chapters on yoga and tai chi

WARM UP

You should warm up your body before any form of physical activity, whether it is sports, gardening or DIY'ing. This prepares the body for action and helps to prevent injuries.

COOL DOWN

Cooling down and stretching after exercise or physical activity is just as important as a warm up. Never "bounce" your stretches and do it gently without pain.

LIFT CORRECTLY

You don't have to lift something heavy in order to hurt your back. Picking up something light incorrectly is far more likely to hurt your back than picking up heavy objects correctly. Lifting things away from your body is also likely to cause damage. When you pick up anything, no matter how heavy, get it as close to your body as you can and keep your back as straight as you can and don't twist with it.

MOVE NOW AND THEN

Whether you are at home, at work or in the car, prolonged sitting causes load on the discs and weakness of the muscles. Get up and move every now and then, even if it is only for a minute. The body is designed for movement not for slouching in front of the TV or driving for hours on end.

GET THE RIGHT FURNITURE

So called "comfortable chairs" do not do your back any good. They are usually too low, too soft and the seat is too long with a rounded back. They force you to slouch and sit awkwardly which puts stress on your back. Choose a chair that is supportive, allows you to sit up correctly with your feet flat on the floor. The right bed is also important. Beds can be too hard. The base of the bed should be firm and the mattress should be soft enough to mould to the contours of your body but be firm enough to give you support in the right places. Futons are not good for most backs and the word "Orthopaedic" when applied to beds means absolutely nothing.

SLEEP PROPERLY

Sleep in a comfortable position. On your side in the "foetal" position is usually the least stressful on your back. Sleeping on your front puts most stress on your back and neck and can lead to trouble. Using a pillow of the right height which supports the neck is also important.

USE MEDICATION WISELY

All drugs have side effects so they should be used wisely. The use of pain killers (paracetamol, cocodomol etc.) and non steroidal anti-inflammatory drugs (nurofen, brufen, diclofenac etc.) only helps to mask the symptoms and not to sort out the problem. Some medication can cause side effects and symptoms that mimic those caused by spine problems. If you want to change your medication please consult your doctor. Pharmacists can also review your medication and make recommendations to your doctor.

CONSULT A SPINAL HEALTH THERAPIST

If you have a long term problem, whether it is just "niggly" or disabling, or if you have a recurring problem, then spinal health care can probably help. Our spinal health therapists can usually give you marked relief from pain and discomfort and improved quality of life as well as decreasing the likelihood of a recurrence.

IV

Physical Stresses

"I'm concerned about the future of football, because we have paid a lot of attention to concussions. We are more aware of concussions. But it's really the repetitive minor injuries, the ones that are asymptomatic that occur on almost every play of the game, the sub-concussive hits: that's the big problem for football. "

Ann McKee

14

Simple Exercises to Strengthen Your Spine

Doing a set of exercises on a regular basis can relieve some causes of spine pain. Exercises can also help strengthen the abdominal and leg muscles so that your lower body can better support your back.

An exercise program or plan can be organised based on the condition that causes the problem. You will need the recommendation of your spinal therapist to come up with an exercise routine that will suit your body's conditions. We would include specific exercises as part of your spinal rehabilitation program

The following are simple exercises that you can try:

Caution - If these cause any pain or other symptoms stop and check with your spinal therapist

Daily Stretches to Improve Spinal Flexibility

Standing Side Bend

- Stand with feet hip width apart
- Let arms hang by side
- Starting at the top of your neck bend your spine sideways
- Work down your spine to the base
- Stack up to the top of your neck
- Repeat to the opposite side
- Repeat 5 times

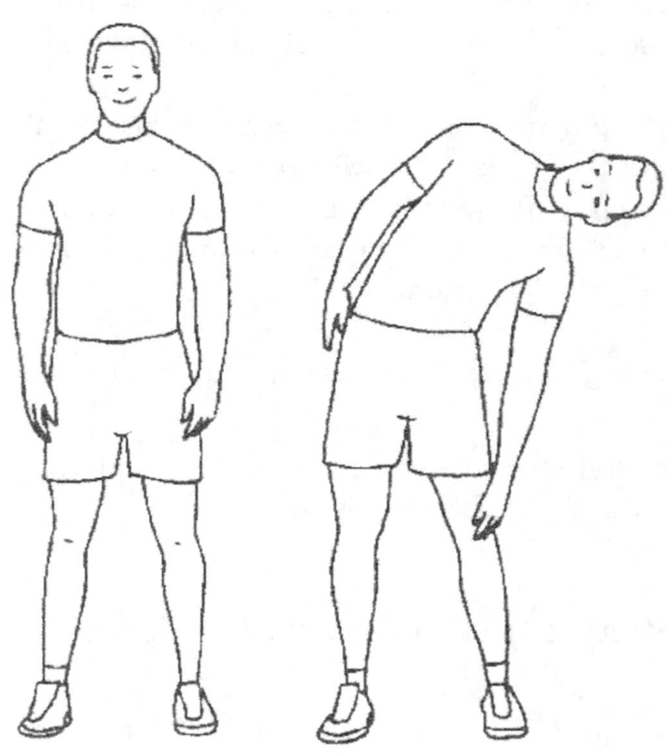

Standing Side Bend

Flexion/Extension

- Stand with feet hip width apart
- Let arms hang by side
- Starting at the top of your neck bend your spine forwards
- Work down your spine to the base
- Stack up to the top of your neck
- Repeat backwards
- Repeat 5 times

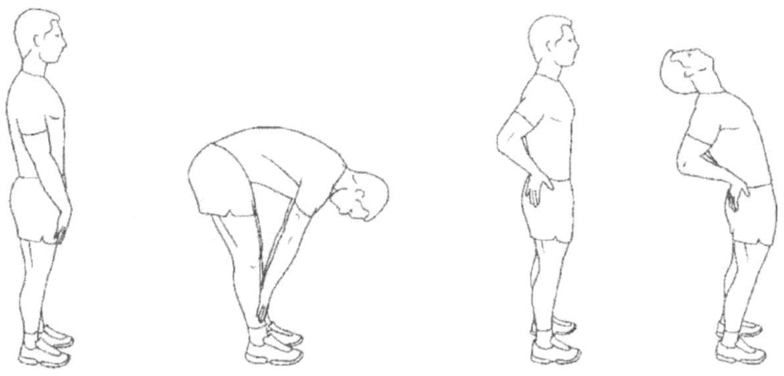

Flexion/Extension

Standing Side Twist

- Stand with feet hip width apart
- Let arms hang by side
- Rotate to the right

- Involve your whole spine and hips
- Repeat to the opposite side
- Repeat 5 times

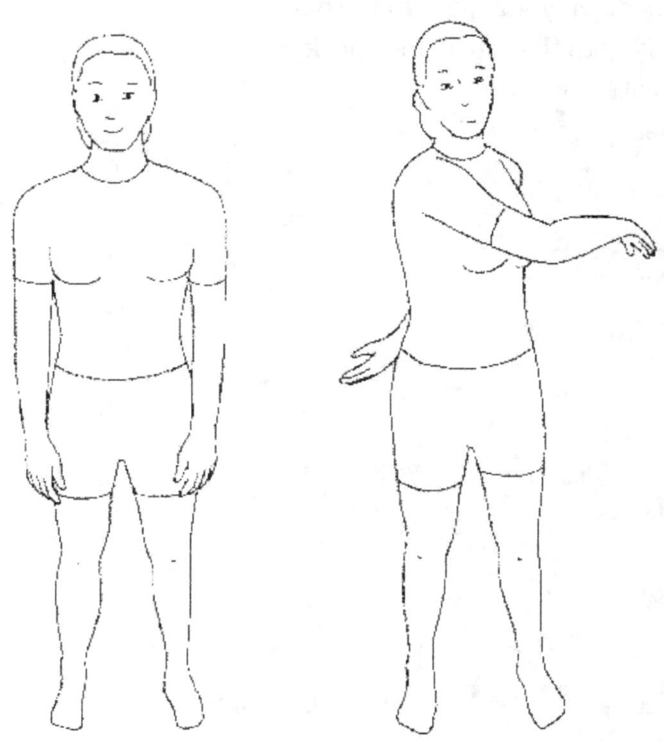

Standing Side Twist

To see these exercises on video use your smart phone to scan the QR code or go online to http://bit.ly/flexibilityysh or http://bit.ly/corestability ysh

Stretches

Core Strength

Exercises to Stabilise Your Spine

Back Lift Lying on Front

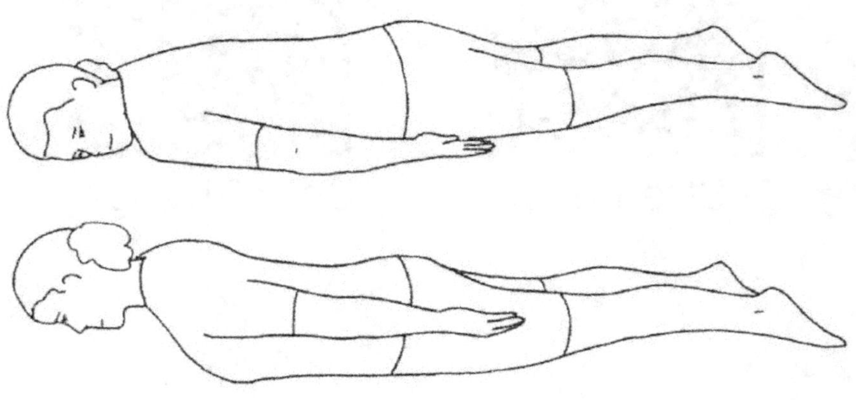

Back Lift Lying on Front

Lie face down with your arms by your sides. Squeeze your buttocks together, contract your back muscles and raise your upper body and arms off the floor. Do this exercise 15 times

Sitting Cross Legged Position

Sit in a cross legged position. Keep the back straight and lean backwards on the arms. Lift upwards and inwards with the pelvic floor muscles. do this 15 times.

Supine Hip Twist

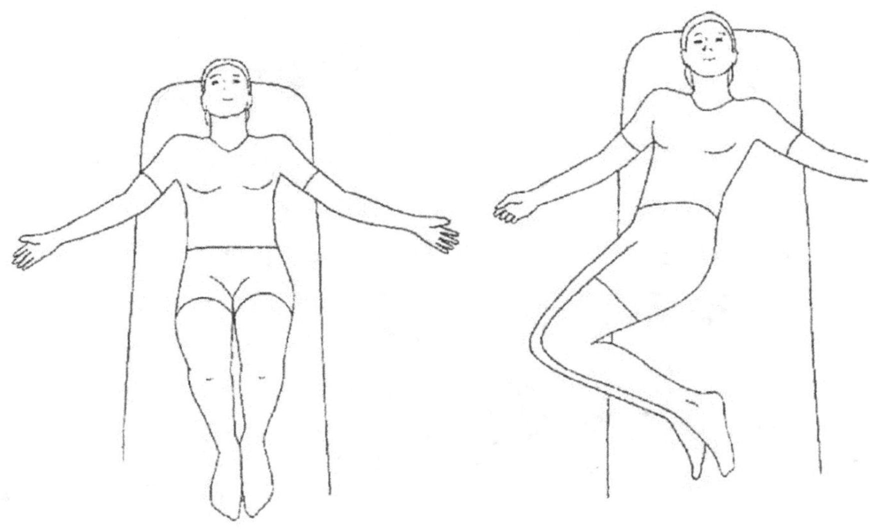

Supine Hip Twist

Lie on your back with your feet on the floor and your hands out to the side. Place your palms downward and keep your legs together. Allow your legs to fall to the side in a controlled motion, using your stomach muscles to lift them up again while keeping your lower back pressed down on the mat. Do this 15 times on each leg.

Press-Up Back Extensions

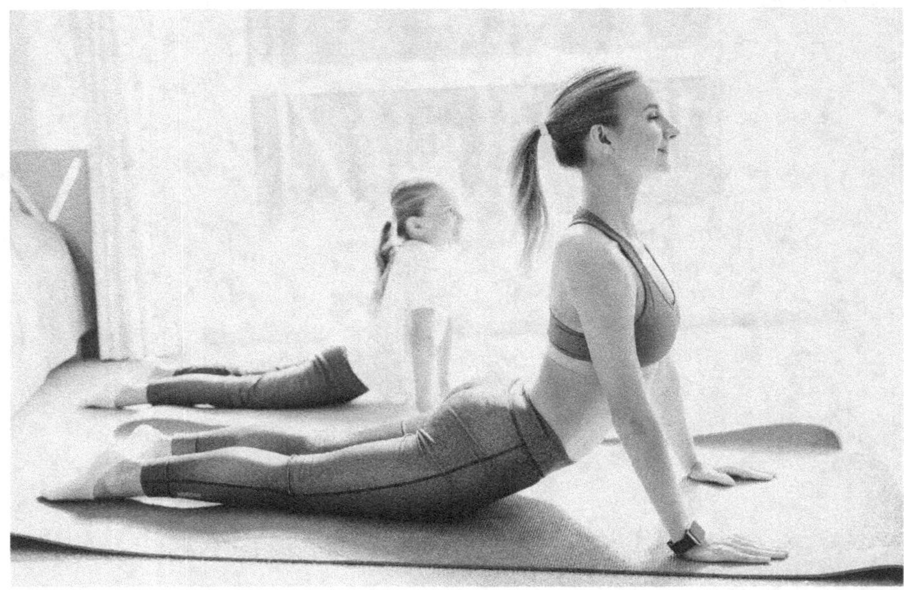

Press–Up Back Extensions

- Lie on your stomach and position your hands under your shoulders.
- Lift your shoulders off the floor by pushing up with your hands.
- Keep your stomach in contact with the floor so it's only your upper back that is lifted up.
- While lifting your shoulders up, try to place your elbows right below them if tolerable.
- Hold the position for 5 seconds or more as tolerated.

Knee Chest Bend

This knee to chest exercise will strengthen your back and abdominal muscles.

- Lie back down on the floor with your knees flexed or bent and your feet flat on the floor.
- Bring one knee towards your chest by bending at the hip while keeping the other knee and leg in the start position.
- Keep your back pressed against the floor and hold the position for about 15 seconds or more as tolerated.
- Repeat this move up to 4 times for each leg.

Pelvic Tilts

Exercises like pelvic tilts help stabilise the spine because of the contracting and relaxing movements of the hip, back and abdominal muscles.

- Lie back on the floor with your knees flexed and your feet flat on the floor.
- Gradually tighten your abdominal muscles and hold for about 10 seconds then relax. This movement makes the pelvis or hips rock back and forth while your back is lying flat on the floor.
- Repeat this up to 10 times. Breathe in and out while performing each movement.

Bridging

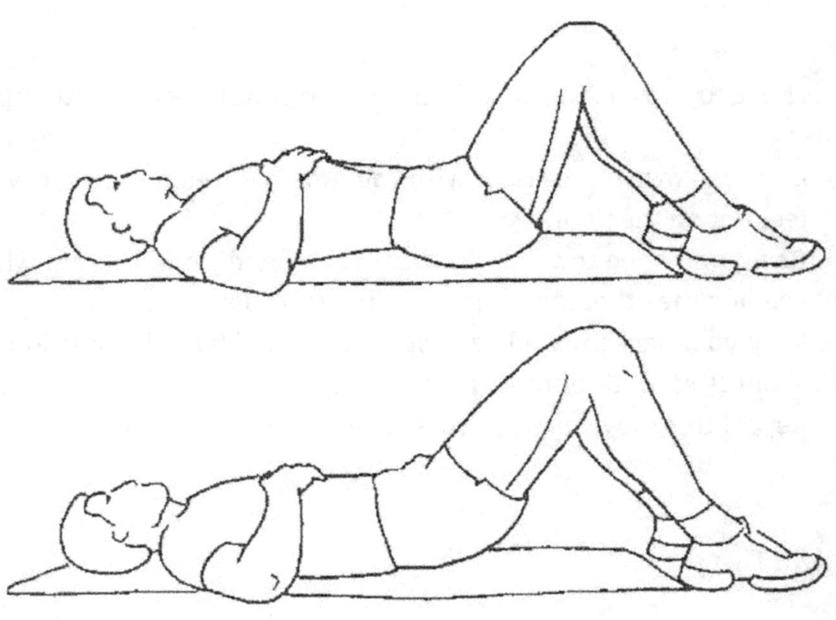

Bridging

Bridging is also one of those exercises that effectively help strengthen your leg and back muscles at the same time.

- Lie down on your back with your knees flexed and only the heels of your feet resting on the floor.
- Press your heels on the floor, tighten your hips and butt, and try to lift your hips off the floor.
- Lift up until your knees, hips, and shoulders are aligned in a straight diagonal line but don't arch your back by tightening your abdominal muscles while lifting.
- Hold the position for about 6 seconds before slowly lowering your back down. Rest for 10 seconds.
- Repeat the movement up to 10 times.

Other exercises that can help improve your body's overall health are aerobic exercises and some Pilates exercises. It is important to consult with your therapist about the exercises that will help your condition and also the exercises that can worsen the problem. If you are unsure how to execute some exercise moves, it is recommended that you consult with a professional coach or trainer than trying out moves at your own risk. This will help you establish a routine for your exercises and keep you motivated.

15

Watch Your Posture

Pay Attention to Your Posture

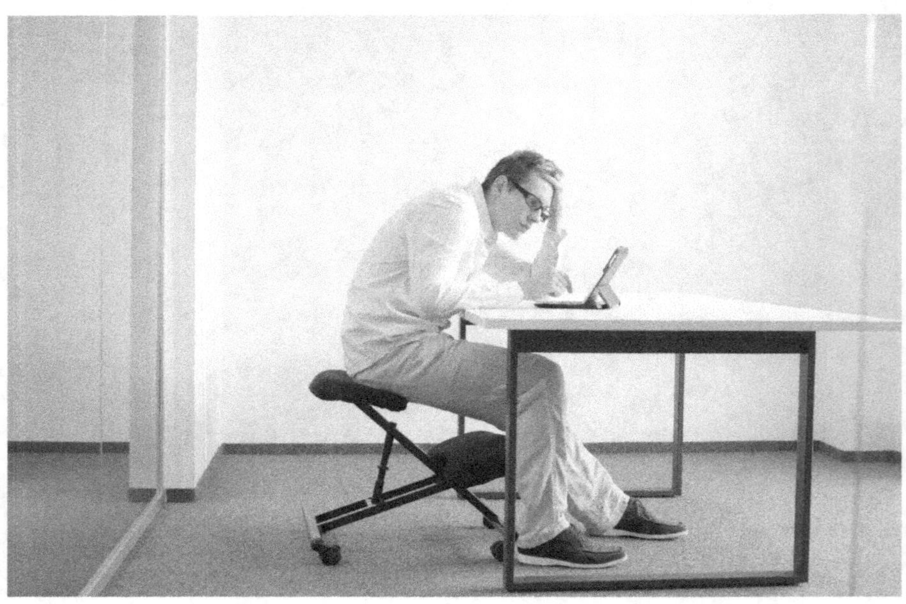

It's a basic rule of thumb that good posture can save you from a lot of
pain. Improper posture often becomes the cause of back pain and knee

pain. Standing up straight is a good way to keep your knees, legs and back safe from stress.

When you slouch, you increase the stress on your joints. As mentioned above, the closer your knees are to the ground, the more stress they bear. So when you stand, make sure there is no incline and you are straight to minimise stress on your knee joint.

Whatever you do, it's important to have proper posture to keep your back muscles and knee joint safe. For example, if you are a student and you need to hold your backpack for a long time, sling it over both your shoulders rather than just one. This divides the stress instead of concentrating it only on one side.

Likewise, if you carry a handbag, keep changing your arms after a few minutes. Don't sling it only on one shoulder for a long time as that can damage the joints in the region.

Proper posture is essential because it also keeps your bones and joints aligned. When you have a bad posture, this alignment gets disturbed and causes the joints to rub against each other. When this keeps happening over time, wear and tear starts to take place.

Your spine takes the stress and starts presenting issues. If you have a kind of job where you need to sit for many hours, make sure you have proper posture. Shoulders should be over hips and you should have good lower back support. Your computer screen should be at eye level so that you don't have to put strain on your neck to look at the screen. Keep your elbows at 90 degrees and the pens or other things you may need should be in easy reach.

When you have to tie your shoe lace, sit on a chair and keep your foot on the opposite knee. In this way, you won't have to bend too far down.

Bending too far increases stress on your joints. So, the idea behind proper posture and exercise is not only to keep joints healthy but also to slow down the degradation process.

Forward Head Posture

Forward head posture increases the strain on many of the muscles attached to the neck which have the job of holding up the head. Over time, forward head posture can lead to muscle imbalances as the body tries to adapt and find efficient ways to hold the head up for straight-ahead vision. Some muscles become elongated and weakened, whereas other muscles become shorter and tighter.

The forward positioning of the head and neck places additional stress on the discs, vertebrae, and facet joints, which increases spinal degeneration. Additionally, as the bottom of the neck flexes forward and the top of the neck over extends in the opposite direction, the spinal canal lengthens through the neck, which increases stretching and tension on the spinal cord and nearby nerve roots.

Use the exercises I show later in this book to gently work on the muscles, ligaments and bones in your neck.

Stop looking down at your computer, phone, knitting or book where possible by changing the position of the work.

Your neck position while sleeping is also important - see the section on choosing a bed.

How to Sit at Your Desk

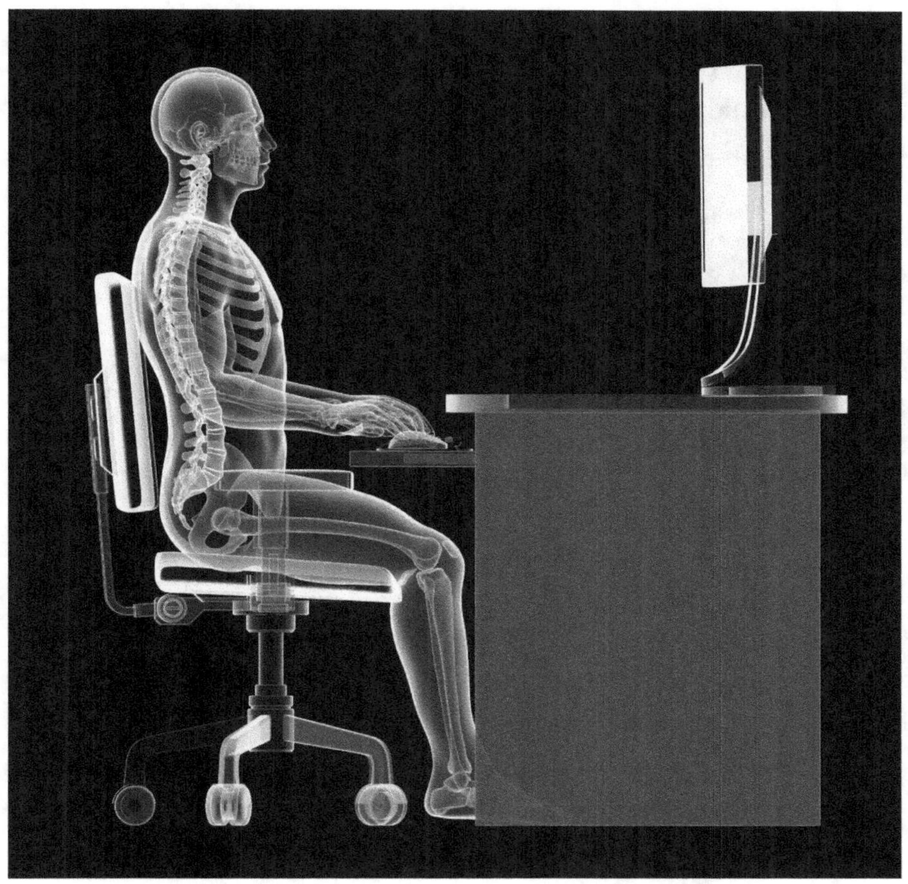

How should I sit at my desk?

Go through the following checklist, and see if you need to correct your posture.

- Your eyes should be level with the top of your computer monitor. This is easier with desktop PCs, but a struggle with laptops where the keyboard and screen are fixed close together. Try a sloping

laptop stand.
- Your shoulders should be relaxed and low, not high and hunched up. You should feel like you're not lifting your shoulders.
- Your fore arms should be parallel to the floor. They should rest on a support, rather than being held up.
- You shouldn't be reaching too far for your keyboard and mouse. You should be able to control them easily with arms bent at the elbow.
- Your feet should be flat on the floor. Just putting your toes on the floor isn't enough!
- Your upper back should be straight. Your lower back has a natural curve that should be supported by your chair.
- You shouldn't slouch in your chair. Your hips should be as close to the back of the chair as possible.
- Your upper legs should be at a 100° angle from your body. Tilt the seat forward or add a seat wedge. This makes easier to keep the proper curves in your spine and reduces fatigue. If you're short, this may mean that you need a footrest. If you're particularly tall, you'll need a higher chair (and may also require a higher desk).
- You should be sitting up straight and your screen should be a full arm's length away from you.
- You shouldn't be leaning to one side. It can be tempting to rest on one arm, but this causes your spine to curve.
- Make sure you are not constantly looking from your desk to the screen or off to one side,
- Don't wedge your phone under your chin while using the computer or taking notes. This can damage your neck or even cause strokes! Use a headset if necessary.

How to Lift Safely

Follow these tips to avoid damaging your spine when you are lifting:
- **Keep a wide base of support.** Your feet should be shoulder-width apart, with one foot slightly ahead of the other.
- **Squat** down, bending at the hips and knees only.
- **Keep good posture.** Look straight ahead, and keep your back straight, your chest out, and your shoulders back. This helps keep your upper back straight while having a slight arch in your lower back.
- **Slowly lift** by straightening your hips and knees (not your back). Keep your back straight, and don't twist as you lift.
- **Hold** the load as close to your body as possible, at the level of your belly button.
- **Use your feet** to change direction, taking small steps.
- **Lead with your hips** as you change direction. Keep your shoulders in line with your hips as you move.
- **Set down** your load carefully, squatting with the knees and hips only.
- Never lift a heavy object above shoulder level.
- Avoid turning or twisting your body while lifting or holding a heavy object

16

Choosing a Bed

Choosing a bed should be easy right? You just get an orthopaedic mattress if you have back problems. However, according to research in the UK, the majority of orthopedic mattresses are too hard, and as a result, only 6% of experts would recommend an orthopedic mattress.

What you are looking for is a bed mattress that is firm and supportive, as opposed to being hard. You should also consider changing your bed more frequently, because older beds and mattresses are less likely to give you the support and comfort that you need.

There would also be an argument here for spending as much money as you can afford on your next bed because it does seem from all available research that sleeping on a high-quality bed can make a significant difference to your spinal health as well as the quality of your sleep.

There is not one ideal sleeping solution that covers everyone. For this reason, you must be willing to do a little research when you buy your next bed. That bed could be the difference between your continuing to suffer spinal health problems for as long as you sleep in it, or solving your problems.

No matter where you live, your local bed store will offer dozens of choices, but do not be persuaded by a sales person to take the bed that they believe is best for your back problems.

Find beds that seem to have the appropriate degree of firmness and support, and test every one for at least 10 minutes in your normal sleeping position. Do this and your back will very soon tell you whether you are looking at the right bed or not!

A quick way to check firmness is to lay on your back and trying to slide your flat hand under the small of your back. If your hand goes in easily the mattress is too hard. If you can't slide it in at all the mattress is too soft. If you can slide your hand in with some difficulty it is about right.

Is the bed the right height for you to get in and out without any back pain or discomfort? If it is so low or so high that entry and exit are likely to stress your spine, you should move on to the next option immediately.

Buy as big a bed as you can afford, particularly if there are two people going to share it. This ensures that you or both of you have plenty of room to move, which should help with a good night's sleep.

Finally, do take time to consider the pillows that you use, and how many of them you generally sleep with. If your pillows are too high, they could significantly alter the shape and angle of your body during sleep, and if your shape is not good, this could offset the benefits that you hope to gain by getting a new bed in the first place.

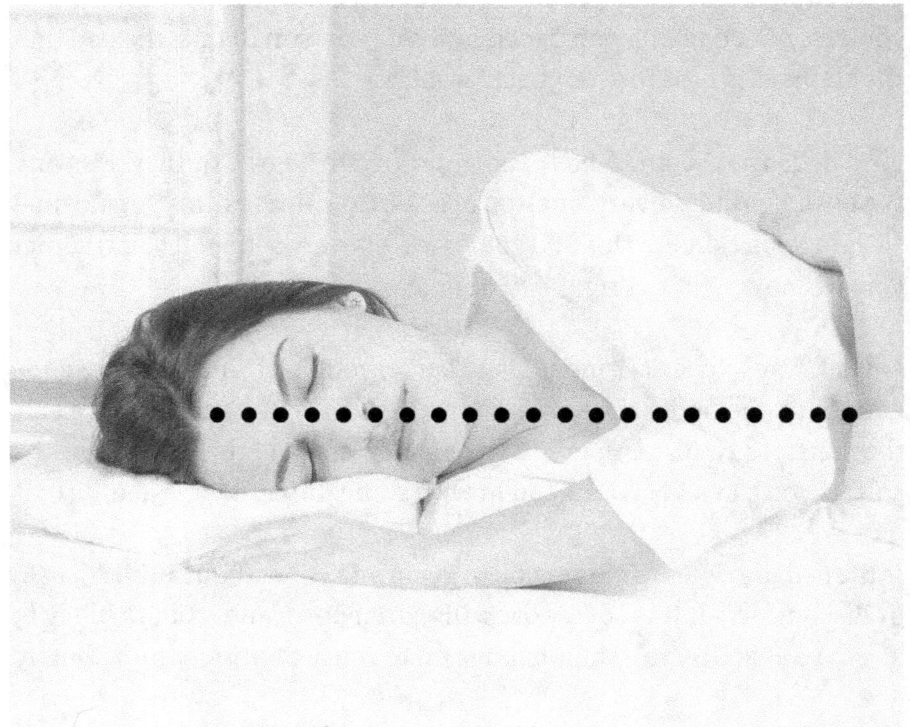

The correct bed and pillows will keep your spine in a neutral position

Also, think about your individual sleeping position, and try to find one that appears to put the least strain on your back. The worst position is to sleep on your front as that puts a lot of twists into your spine.

17

Yoga, Tai Chi, Pilates or Dancing to Improve Your Spinal Health

It is important to gently exercise all the joints in your spine to keep them supple and to keep the muscles and other structures around them working properly.

If you don't use it you lose it!

The benefits of yoga, pilates and tai chi are that, done properly, they gently exercise all of the joints in your spine. They are low-impact, meaning that they won't cause damage to the joints by putting excessive load on them or causing rapid changes in direction. Yoga and tai chi also incorporate elements of meditation which helps with stress relief.

Certain forms of dance are also very good at gently exercising the spine and relieving stress.

Ballroom dancing is especially useful as the complex movements you have to learn exercise the brain pathways.

Ballet and break dancing tend to be high impact, as do some forms of modern dance.

Whatever you choose it would also be highly advisable to start training under the professional supervision of a suitably qualified teacher. While you can follow online courses, it will certainly be safer and probably more productive for you to learn properly from the outset and you will also get the benefits from the social interactions.

Also bear in mind that each trainer has developed their own style. It is important to talk to the trainer before you start to find out if their style is right for you.

Yoga

Yoga is not simply a form of exercise or something that is only focused on striking certain poses. Yoga is focused on teaching devotees to adopt a total balanced approach to life, taking in both physical exercise and mental adaptability and adroitness.

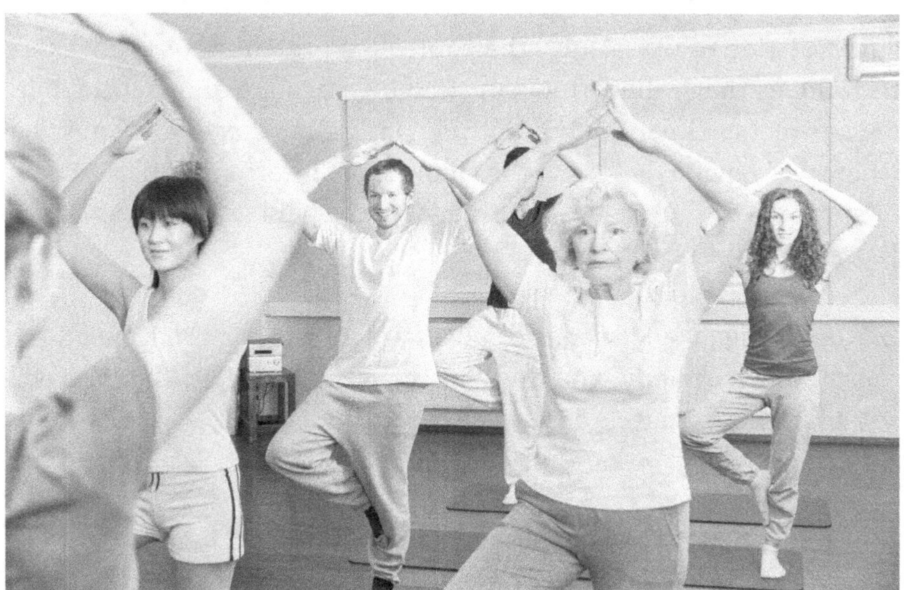

Most importantly for your spinal health, yoga lays great emphasis on body alignment, and it is often the fact that people's bodies are forced into badly aligned positions that causes symptoms in the first place.

For example, if you spend many hours everyday sitting at your desk working on a computer, or behind the wheel of your car driving, you are putting your body into a position which is almost inevitably going to cause stress to develop in your back. Consequently, even though there is no one single event or situation that causes you to suffer back pain, the daily misalignment of your body is inevitably going to cause back problems eventually.

There are many reasons why yoga is likely to be far more effective as a form of exercise for alleviating or reducing your back when compared to other forms of exercise.

In the first place, because yoga places a great deal of emphasis on the spiritual side of practicing, the controlled breathing or pranayama techniques that you learn when studying yoga are an essential part of the practice. Deep, slow breathing naturally relaxes your muscles, which will obviously reduce the chances of suffering a muscle strain or sprain in the first place, and alleviate the pain if you have already caused a strain.

On top of this, yogic asanas or poses are all about stretching all the muscles in your body, and this also makes it less likely that you will suffer strains or muscle damage in the future.

Tai Chi

Tai chi is a non-competitive martial art known for its health benefits. As a form of exercise, it combines gentle physical exercise and stretching with mindfulness.

You may have seen videos of groups of elderly Chinese people exercising in the park. They believe that regular tai chi maintains health.

Various research studies suggest the benefits of tai chi might include improved balance, fall prevention, pain management, and cognitive function in people with and without chronic conditions.

Other studies have shown that exercise which includes complex movements and coordination reduce the risk of dementia and Alzheimers. Tai chi is one of those exercises along with dancing.

Other possible benefits include improved sleep quality and an enhanced immune system.

Pilates

Plagued by asthma and rickets as a child, Joseph Pilates created an exercise method which sprang from his determination to strengthen his frail and sickly body. He studied yoga, martial arts, Zen meditation and Greek and Roman exercises.

In general, Pilates uses a combination of approximately 50 simple, repetitive exercises to create muscular exertion. Exercises can be adapted to provide either gentle strength training for rehabilitation or a strenuous workout. There is a wide variation in the approaches taken so talk to the instructor before taking a class to make sure it is right for you.

The exercises are designed to increase muscle strength and endurance, as well as flexibility and to improve posture and balance.

V

Chemical Stresses

*"If we could give every individual the right amount of
nourishment and exercise, not too little and not too much,
we would have the safest way to health."*

Hippocrates

18

Nutrition

To repair your body you need to send the right materials to the right places in the right order.

- If your nervous system is compromised you won't know fully where the damage is and where and when you should send the materials.
- If your diet is poor you won't have the right materials to send to the right places.

If either the nerve supply or the nutrient supply (or both) are reduced in quality healing may be slower or incomplete.

Under Nutrition

You are not taking in enough of the right materials

Over Nutrition

You are taking in too much food (even if it is the right sort). Your body can't use it all and has to expend energy storing it in fat cells for potential use in times of famine.

This puts extra stress on the spine because of the extra weight you are carrying, but also puts stress on the body systems responsible for processing the food.

Toxicity

You are taking in materials which are toxic to the body. These materials can't be used productively in repairing or building the body. Instead they cause stress to the toxin elimination systems of the body and the body has to waste energy trying to clear out the toxins.

Toxins in food can include artificial additives, colourings and flavourings, and processed foods such as highly refined sugars. They can also include residues from pesticides, hormones and other chemicals used in food production and toxins that are building up in the environment such as dioxins and micro particles of plastic.

(According to the nonprofit organization Environmental Working Group, the average newborn baby has 287 known toxins in his or her umbilical cord blood. https://drhyman.com/blog/2010/05/19/is-there-toxic-waste-in-your-body-2/)

Toxins can also come into your body through the air, through chemicals on the skin (some beauty products for example), smoking, alcohol, drugs (medical and illegal)

Food Intolerance

We use a company called Cambridge Nutritional Sciences (www.cam-nutri.com) to test for food intolerances if our clients are showing signs of chronic inflammation.

A food intolerance is different from a food allergy.

A **food allergy** is technically known as a Type I immediate IgE hyper-sensitivity immune response and this reaction typically occurs very quickly (within minutes to hours) after eating an offending food, with symptoms ranging from mild to severe.

A **food intolerance** can happen if food components in patients with increased intestinal permeability (leaky gut syndrome) enter the blood-stream from the intestinal lumen on a continuous basis so the immune mechanisms undergo constant activation. The body produces IgG antibodies which can build up. This can eventually overload the immune system's ability to clear such complexes efficiently, which results in chronic inflammation.

Because a food intolerance builds up over time and you don't respond immediately to a food it is difficult to work out what is going on. The quickest way to find out if you have a food intolerance and which foods to avoid is to have an IgG blood test.

Balance Your Diet

If you don't lead a healthy life with a balanced diet, health issues will catch up with you sooner than you'd like. There's always room for improvement and you can start making changes in your diet at any point in life. A joint-healthy diet helps keep away pain, stiffness and reduced mobility.

Nutrients that Nourish Your Joints

The food you eat contains different nutrients such as fats, proteins, fiber, vitamins and carbohydrates. The two most important nutrients for joint health are minerals and vitamins.

The most notable among these is perhaps **calcium** which keeps your bones strong and can prevent osteoporosis. But while many people give calcium the credits it deserves for bone and joint health, they often forget about **magnesium**. However, the truth is that calcium needs to be paired with magnesium, and even **vitamin D** to be most effective.

You need to have a good balance of all three as each is dependent on the other for optimal performance. For instance, while calcium promotes bone density, magnesium assists the transport of calcium across cell membranes. At the same time, magnesium promotes enzymes that convert vitamin D to its active form, which, in turn helps the body absorb calcium better.

Magnesium also plays a role in strengthening bones and maintaining cartilage. It also regulates nerve and muscle function, ensuring that everything is under control. Studies have shown that magnesium prevents degradation of bones and increases bone density. It's also been found to be effective against postmenopausal osteoporosis.

People with joint issues often suffer from low levels of vitamin D as well. According to studies, Vitamin D seems to ward off conditions like osteomalacia or soft bones, or osteoporosis, resulting in loss of bone mass. Supplementing well with this vitamin may help you take better care of your bones and joints.

Another vitamin that deserves attention in this area is **vitamin C**. as one of the most powerful antioxidants, it can help prevent oxidative stress in the body. Oxidative stress also harms the synovial membrane in joints causing the synovial fluid to leak, compromising joint lubrication. Here vitamin C can provide cushion and lubrication to the area by preventing oxidative damage.

Best Foods for Joint Health

Naturally, the best foods for joint health will include these aforementioned nutrients along with others. If you already suffer from joint-related conditions, then altering your diet may actually help reduce your painful or discomforting issues.

For instance, there are some foods that can actually help reduce the effects of arthritis and also relieve pain. Many patients suffering from arthritis admit that changes in their diet plan have helped reduce the severity of their symptoms.

One of the best foods to eat if you have painful or inflamed joints is fatty fish. Salmon and sardines are rich in **omega 3 fatty acids**. Omega 3s reduce inflammation in the body and it has been found that in the presence of this fatty acid, the amount of inflammatory mediators is also low in the body.

Incorporating Omega 3s in your diet will reduce morning stiffness, provide pain-relief and cool down your body. These fatty acids are especially helpful for people with rheumatoid arthritis.

Garlic is also very important for people suffering from painful joints. Its immune strengthening properties make cells stronger and can target inflammation as well. By lowering the amount of inflammatory markers in the body, garlic helps lessen the pain associated with arthritis and similar conditions.

Likewise, **ginger** is also very effective in reducing pain from knee arthritis. A very easy way to incorporate these two foods in your diet is to make a garlic ginger paste and use it for flavoring in your meals.

Broccoli is not only effective for keeping your weight in check but also great for joint health. It's involved in blocking a certain type of cell that accelerates the progression of rheumatoid arthritis. **Walnuts** are also anti-inflammatory in their effect and they may even reduce the need for painkillers. If you love **berries**, then you are in luck because berries also reduce inflammatory markers associated with arthritis. Whether it's black berries or strawberries, all kinds are great for joint health.

Spinach is another green that helps promote joint health. Spinach is a powerful green vegetable that helps prevent the progression of osteoarthritis. At the same time, it also improves cartilage health and reduces inflammatory agents that cause rheumatoid arthritis. Another fruit for fighting joint pain is **Grapes**. The outer covering of grapes contains reseveratrol, which has antioxidant properties. Grapes also slow down the thickening of joints and block the production of cells causing rheumatoid arthritis. You can also prepare your meals in **olive oil** to promote the health of your joints.

Foods to Avoid

There are some foods that you need to avoid in order to prevent progression or worsening of joint pains. Firstly, **fried foods** and **processed foods** are a huge No for anyone with painful joints. These foods can significantly decrease the body's immunity and cause inflammation.

When you cut down the intake of such foods, the body's natural defense system gets restored. Instead of eating frozen foods, cook at home and try to go for greens and fruits. Even foods cooked at high temperatures can make your body more prone to arthritis, so opt for more suitable recipes.

AGE or Advanced Glycation End Product, as they increase in the body, can cause inflammation. These are produced when you eat grilled or heated foods. The body activates cytokines that cause inflammation in response, to fight these compounds. As a result of that, the overall level of inflammation increases in the body causing a risk of joint pain or deterioration. Cut down on these foods so that blood AGE levels can be low.

You might love nibbling on cheese slices but this isn't healthy for your joints. **Dairy products** contribute to joint deterioration due to their protein content. Proteins present in dairy products can irritate the surrounding tissue of joints in many people. You can get the same proteins from other sources without the side effects, so it's advised to switch to a restricted dairy diet.

Corn oil is present in many snacks and some baked goods too. It gives a pleasant taste to food but can trigger inflammatory markers to go in action and increases the risk of joint pain. This is because corn oil is rich in Omega 6 fatty acids. Instead of eating omega 6s, you can try using oils rich in Omega 3s, such as olive oil and flaxseed oil.

Some cuts of **red meat** can also exacerbate inflammation as they are rich in saturated fats. Also, excessive consumption of red meat can cause obesity which is another factor contributing to joint pain. Experts say that gluten can also cause inflammation in people who are already suffering from an autoimmune disease such as rheumatoid arthritis.

Although **alcohol** doesn't really count as food, increased intake can lead to deterioration of joint health. A controlled amount of alcohol can actually prevent rheumatoid arthritis but the problem begins when you start drinking too much of it.

Overconsumption of alcohol leads to production of a protein called C – reactive protein which is a signal for inflammation. So, it can worsen the cases of rheumatoid arthritis. Balancing your diet is the first step towards improving joint health.

If you would like to explore the science of nutrition and weight loss in more detail I have produced an online course https://www.onboard101.com/weightlossscience101

19

Lose weight and get fitter

Watch Your Weight

So now that you know that one of the factors affecting joint health is lack of physical activity, what do you do about it? Well, you naturally start off with some form of exercise to improve joint flexibility and range of motion. But at the same time, you also have to watch your weight.

When your body becomes too heavy to be supported by your joints and bones, problems start to arise. As such, you need to exercise and eat right to keep your body at an optimal weight.

How Weight Affects Joints

If you have a sensation of pain when walking for a while or climbing up the stairs, then you should take a look at your weight. Being overweight increases your chances of getting osteoarthritis. As mentioned earlier, this condition is caused by the wear and tear in joints and is the most common form of bone degradation.

When you're overweight, there's extra stress on the joints that bear your weight. The most common of these joints is the knee joint and it's the first one to get affected by excess weight. The second reason why weight is detrimental for joints is that as your weight increases, the inflammatory markers in the body also increase. This further causes joint deterioration in other places such as your hands and neck.

The extra pounds in your body stressing your joints can lead to degeneration of cartilage and joint damage. In cases of osteoporosis, being overweight also increases the rate of bone degeneration. By shedding weight, you can protect your joints from extra stress and any further damage. Experts suggest that you should lose about 10% of your body weight and then see if the symptoms improve.

If they do, then it's your weight causing the problems in the first place. Obesity further reduces any physical activity which becomes another cause for joint issues in the long run. And if you already suffer from an extreme case of arthritis, high endurance exercise can also damage to your joints.

So, it's important to get guidance from an expert about the kind of exercises you can and should do. In osteoarthritis, sitting for extended periods of time causes stress on the joints and worsens the pain. If you have an office job, make a habit to take a walk or do short exercises after every hour.

Reduce Stress on Joints

Weight loss is a great way to reduce stress on your joints. On average, the amount of pressure or stress on your knees is 1 ½ times that of your body weight. So, if you weigh 300 pounds, you are putting 450 pounds of stress on your knees. This is when you are in standing position. As the incline increases, the stress increases too.

As such, when you climb stairs, there's more stress on your knees. If your knees are extremely close to the ground, like when you tie a shoelace, the weight increases to three or four times of your body weight. Experts say that just a 10 pound increase in weight increase 30 to 40 pounds of stress on your joints. The joints work fine while they are still young and healthy but after an extended period of time, they give up.

So just imagine that if you lose weight, how much stress you'll be able to reduce on your knees. When you're young, the body's cells proliferate at a considerable rate. With age, this process slows down so the damaged cells don't get repaired as quickly as they did during your youth.

So start slow and you'll be able to lose the extra pounds very easily. Physical activity in the form of exercise is a proven way of slowing the progression of arthritis. Just like any machine, the body wears away if it is not being used properly. So, put your muscles and joints to use so that they do not rot away.

Every pound you lose represents about 3500 calories. So, if you're hoping to lose one pound in a week, you need to burn about 500 calories in a day. The exercise plan you follow must at least help you lose 500 calories in a day.

Along with exercise, you also need to focus on your diet. Even if you're young and not arthritic, it's essential that you watch your weight to dodge this disease in a few years' time.

20

Home Remedies for Easing Joint Pain

Doctors often prescribe painkillers and anti-inflammatory drugs for joint pain. But if you're someone concerned about the side effects of medication, you may just wish to use some tried-and-true home remedies instead. Where the pain isn't too bad or too frequent, you may be able to get relief from these simple home remedies. These remedies are effective for treating joint pain in knees, neck, hips, ankles and lower back.

Epsom Salts

Epsom salts have been used traditionally for treating joint and muscle pains. These salts are rich in sulphates and magnesium, like many supplements used for treating joint pain. They can be administered topically as they are absorbed by the skin. These salts aid in relaxing the tensed regions of the body while keeping muscle spasms at minimum. You can simply add two cups of Epsom salts to your bath water and stay in it for about half an hour.

Or, you can make a compress of these salts and apply to the skin topically. For doing this, add two cups of Epsom salts in one gallon of water to form a dilute mixture. Then dip a towel or face cloth in this solution and apply to the affected area. Adding essential oils to the mixture can increase the benefits of this remedy.

Essential Oils

Essential oils are also great home remedies for joint pain. Lavender essential oil is extremely helpful in treating those conditions in which the pain is already present and is worsening. If you take an Epsom salt bath, simply add a few drops of lavender oil to the water. If the affected area is swollen and feels warm, this could be a case of bursitis. Apply peppermint oil to the area. The cooling menthol effect of this oil will reduce the swelling and inflammation.

Eucalyptus essential oil also reduces inflammation associated with arthritis and osteoarthritis. Along with that, it also helps prevent edema or fluid retention. Turmeric oils are not commonly available in many areas but they are helpful in reducing joint pain that occurs due to osteoarthritis, rheumatoid arthritis and bursitis. You can also add more turmeric to your daily meals to get maximum benefits.

Soaking In The Sun

You'd be surprised at how helpful a good sun bath can be in getting rid of pain. Many people with joint issues have such complaints because of lower levels of Vitamin D. Your body naturally produces Vitamin D when you go out in the sun. Expose your body to the sun for 20 minutes three to four times a week. Even this much exposure is enough for your body to make enough Vitamin D. So whenever it's a nice day outside, take a walk by yourself or with a friend and do your joints a huge favor.

Hot and Cold Packs

Hot and cold packs are probably the most accessible home remedy for joint pain. Both, hot and cold treatments can help relieve pain and stiffness. There are two types of hot treatments; dry and moist. Taking long warm showers will often relieve any stiffness in the joints. Take a warm shower in the morning to feel more energetic during the day.

You can also keep a heated pad on affected areas to loosen up your joints while you sleep. When heat reaches the damaged areas, it provides relief and soothes muscles along with joints.

Cold treatments are great for reducing inflammation and ridding the body of pain. Apply an ice pack to the affected area for quick relief. These two methods are lifesavers when the pain gets worse.

Chamomile Tea Poultice

Chamomile tea can also reduce the pain associated with arthritis. It helps cool down the body and reduce inflammation. There are different inflammatory markers in the body that heat up the system and disturb the internal balance. This tea soothes everything and calms the immune system.

To make a poultice, take four chamomile tea bags and add them in a cup of boiling water. Steep and keep the cup covered for about 20 minutes. Then remove the tea bags from the cup and soak a clean face cloth in the cup. When soaked with the liquid, apply to the affected area and you'll feel instant relief.

Swimming

As odd as it may sound, swimming can actually help reduce the pain that comes with arthritis. It is also a good exercise for losing weight if you suffer from joint pain. High intensity exercise is almost impossible for someone who has painful joints. Instead, exercising in water is easier as it bears less weight.

Not only does swimming reduce pain, it also increases flexibility in the hip region. In addition, it strengthens the hip muscles for increased mobility. In some areas, there are special swimming classes for people who suffer from arthritis. So, look around or go for a swim occasionally.

Soothing Music

If you love listening to music, you can actually use your hobby to get rid of the pain. Studies show that people who listened to soothing music had reduced arthritis pain as compared to people who were not given a music prescription. Besides, music also reduces the depression that comes with joint pain.

You don't necessarily have to listen to a particular genre or kind of music. The important thing is that you enjoy the music. If you like the music, your body activates several hormones that cause pain relief, acting as body's own natural pain killers. Listening to your favourite music for a bit every day can help take down the pain by several notches.

Walking

While this isn't exactly a remedy, it's a good way of keeping pain at bay. Walking barefoot reduces the pressure on joints by 12% as compared to the stress your joints feel when you walk in shoes. When you buy shoes, make sure that they mimic the natural arch of your foot. Lifting up your heel can cause stress on your joints. So, avoid wearing heels daily as this can cause damage to your joints. Wearing heels for extended period of time also increases the risk of joint damage.

21

Best Supplements for Joint Health

Increased friction between joints leads to the sensation of pain and discomfort. While many resort to medication as the primary solution to the problem, supplements are also a popular alternative.

And while there are many supplements available, here we'll only look at some of the best in this category. These supplements have all been backed by scientific research and deemed most effective to addressing joint related issues.

Glucosamine

Glucosamine is a complex carbohydrate found in the body primarily in three different forms; glucosamine sulphate, glucosamine hydrochloride and N-acetyl-glucosamine. Among these, glucosamine sulphate is the most common form and is extracted from the outer covering of shellfish. To treat joint issues, this supplement may be used alone or combined with chondroitin or shark cartilage for added benefits.

The reason why this is considered beneficial for joint health is because it plays a vital role in the formation of cartilage. As you've already seen, cartilage thins and deteriorates with age. If anything, it needs help from supplementation to keep it healthy.

Evidence suggests that glucosamine helps in slowing down this process. It assists cartilage repair and formation by incorporating sulfur into the structure. Likewise, swelling also reduces in the presence of glucosamine. People suffering from hip or knee arthritis can sufficiently benefit from this supplement.

The pain-relieving effect of glucosamine lasts for about 3 months from usage so it may not exactly offer a long-term solution. Results may take a good 6-8 weeks to become noticeable, but will likely be more effective than those achieved by using over-the-counter and prescription medication.

Chondroitin

Chondroitin naturally occurs in the body in bone and cartilage while supplementary chondroitin is extracted from animal cartilage.

Chondroitin is present in the form of chondroitin sulphate and is often administered alongside glucosamine. Its benefits are somewhat similar to that of glucosamine.

This supplement helps the cartilage retain water so that excess rubbing between bones may be prevented. At the same time, it also slows down the progression of osteoarthritis.

When used on its own or in association with other supplements, chondroitin improves the shock-absorbing ability of collagen protein. Also, it inhibits the functioning of enzyme that causes cartilage breakdown.

When used in conjunction with another supplement, hyaluronic acid, the two develop into a spring-like molecule. This improves the elasticity and strength of the cartilage. At the same time, chondroitin sulphate also signals the immune system to prevent cartilage breakdown by increasing collagen synthesis.

Chondroitin is especially beneficial for people with hand arthritis. Although it doesn't enhance grip strength or reduce the need for pain medication, it still alleviates morning stiffness in such individuals.

It can also serve as an alternative for Non Steroidal Anti Inflammatory Drugs (NSAIDS) for people who can't take them as no side effects of this supplement have been reported.

SAM-E

SAM-E is a compound that's naturally formed in the body. It plays a role in synthesis, activation and degradation of hormones, drugs and different proteins. The body produces chemicals that induce inflammatory responses to activate the immune system. SAM-E reduces the activity of these mediators to lower pain in joints.

In osteoarthritis, proteoglycan, which is a constituent of cartilage, doesn't get produced in sufficient amounts. SAM-E enhances the working of enzymes that form proteoglycan to reverse cartilage degradation. SAM-E also plays a role in reducing stiffness in joints. Consequently, mobility is improved. It's been seen to be very helpful in reversing the excessive fatigue and body pain associated with fibromyalgia.

Tendonitis, which refers to the inflammation of tendons in the body, is also treatable with the help of SAM-E. Bursa, a cushioning sac filled with fluid between tendons and bones, can be inflamed. This leads to swelling of the bursa and joint pain.

SAM-E is particularly helpful in reducing swelling and tenderness. Individuals suffering from chronic lower back pain due to weight or sports injury, can also benefit from this supplement.

Capsaicin

Capsaicin is a component of chili peppers. It's the constituent that causes a burning sensation in your mouth because it causes a sting when it comes in contact with any body tissue. The working of capsaicin is quite interesting as it relieves pain by affecting the nerve cells. It's used in form of a topical cream or patch.

It stimulates the activation of certain nerve receptors that are involved in causing itching or stinging sensation. Capsaicin keeps the receptors activated for a long period of time.

After some time, the receptors' ability to function is lost due to over-reception. So, these receptors also stop processing signals for pain induction. When used on regular basis, this supplement helps numb the sensation of pain by overusing the receptors.

Capsaicin is effective in relieving pain that is caused by rheumatoid arthritis, fibromyalgia and osteoarthritis. It is so effective that it can actually help lower the pain by 50% after just a month of usage. It also helps reduce pain which results from nerve damage as a result of diabetic neuropathy or HIV.

Curcumin

Curcumin is a chemical abundantly present in turmeric. Although turmeric is only used as a flavoring agent in cooking or to give color in cosmetics, it also has benefits for joint health. Curcumin reduces pain associated with rheumatoid arthritis and osteoarthritis.

When the bursa swells and causes irritation of joints, curcumin can also aid in reducing swelling and inflammation in the region for smooth cushioning and improved mobility. It blocks the enzymes that are involved in formation of inflammatory mediators in the body.

One of the targets of curcumin is COX-2, a mediator that is also target of many pain-relieving medicines. So, curcumin can act as an alternative to NSAIDS. Instead of reducing joint inflammation, this supplement actually prevents further inflammation. Patients suffering from knee osteoarthritis can benefit from this supplement. In some cases of rheumatoid arthritis, curcumin actually tends to be more effective than NSAIDS.

Omega 3s

Omega 3s are naturally found in fish oils and have been consumed for centuries for their benefits. One of the main benefits of omega 3s is pain relief.

The two important omega 3s for relieving pain are DHA (docosahexaenoic acid) and EPA (eicosapentaenoic acid). Omega 3s have shown most effectiveness in relieving pain due to rheumatoid arthritis. They don't reverse joint damage or play a role in synthesis of new cartilage. Instead, their only function is for pain relief.

When omega 3s are taken as supplements, they get converted to resolvins in the body. These compounds are 10,000 times more effective than normal fatty acids. They inhibit the functioning of immune system mediators that cause inflammation.

For inflammation to occur, the body has its own on and off switch. Omega 3s inhibit the turning on of these switches so that the inflammatory pathway cannot proceed.

Hyaluronic Acid

Hyaluronic acid is a component of synovial fluid which is present between joints and allows easy gliding of bones. In patients with rheumatoid arthritis, this component starts to break up and functioning of the fluid is affected.

While its primary administration is through injections as a pain reliever, the same is also found in small doses in supplements. Research shows that low doses of this acid can reduce chronic pain and joint stiffness, though results may vary from person to person.

You can take hyaluronic acid for knee osteoarthritis in the form of 50mg tablets twice a day with meals. If your case is more severe, your doctor may recommend an injection.

It incorporates into the synovial fluid and reduces friction between the bones. In this way, it reduces stiffness of joints and enhances mobility.

Hyaluronic acid is especially used for the treatment of knee, hip and ankle arthritis as these are the regions where joints are extremely critical. The ball and socket joint in the hips that provide maximum mobility can often be affected due to arthritis. So this supplement helps rebuild the shock-absorbing fluid present in the joints and acts like grease in bones.

Hyaluronic acid injections are prescribed for patients when pain from knee arthritis can no longer be controlled by anti-inflammatory drugs and NSAIDS.

VI

Mental Stresses

"Our bodies are our gardens our wills are our gardeners."

William Shakespeare

22

Manage Stress

How Does Stress Affect Your Spinal Health?

Whole books have been written on the effects of stress on the general health of the body. Here I am going to focus on the direct effects of stress on your spine and nervous system.

Have you ever heard people say things like "I feel wound up", "I feel bitter and twisted", "I've got the weight of the world on my shoulders", "X is a pain in the neck"

When a thought goes through your mind your body always reacts. Normally you wouldn't notice anything and it wouldn't affect your health because it is fleeting. (This is how we can "read" people)

When you are feeling stressed or defensive you go into the stressed posture. Your shoulders come up, you clench your fists and your jaw and your breathing gets faster. You have gone into "fight or flight" mode - you are preparing to start punching or to run away.

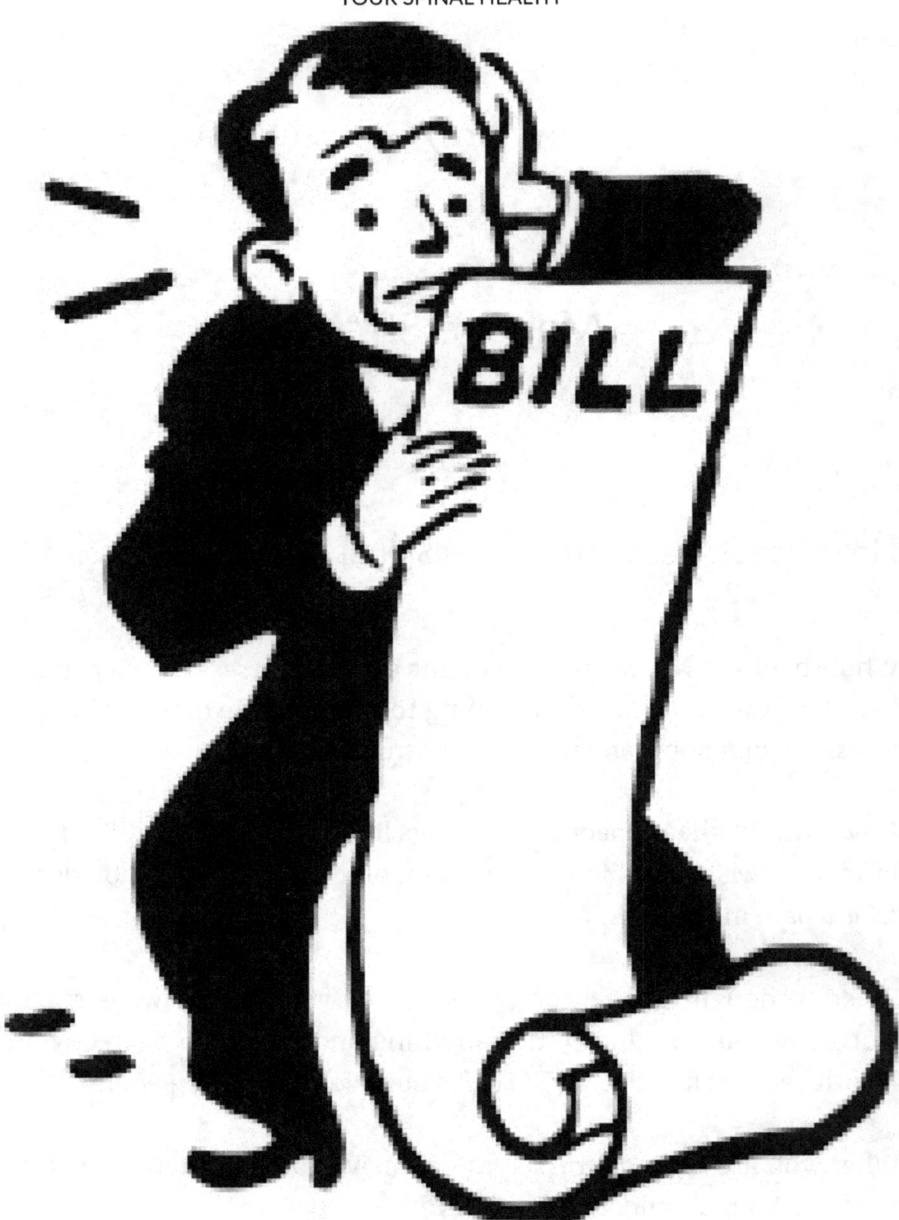

A lot of things in life can cause the stress response

If the stress keeps happening every day or it is constant your body has to change so that it can adapt to it. The stressed posture becomes permanent as your bones, ligaments and muscles grow into the stressed position.

The stressed posture also feeds back into your brain and affects your mood. To see this in action try the following exercise:-

- Drop your head forward, bring your shoulders up and forward and put your face into a frown.
- Now try to feel enthusiastic or happy!
- Not easy is it!

Being a chiropractor over the last 20 years has necessarily meant becoming a life coach as well because if I don't help people to recognise and deal with their stress they keep reverting back to their stressed posture.

I have also found over the years that improving a clients spinal health and posture automatically improves their mood and their ability to deal with stress. Try the following exercise to see this in action:-
- Hold yourself straight, drop your shoulders down, open your chest, breath deeply and look straight ahead.
- Now try to feel depressed or stressed
- Was it harder to feel those negative emotions?

By getting someone straighter and helping them to manage stress we get them into a "virtuous spiral"

And,of course, as your spinal health improves you will experience less pain and be able to do more which will also improve your mood and your ability to deal with life stresses.

A Simple Stress Management Exercise

If you feel yourself getting stressed or feel tense in your shoulders do the following exercise:-
- Breathe in through your nose for a count of 3
- Hold the breath for a count of 1
- Breath out through your mouth until you get to 10

You will notice that you are breathing using your whole chest and your shoulders will drop down and feel less tense.

Two things are happening here:-
1. You are getting more oxygen into your body
2. While you are thinking about your breathing and counting you can't also think about the stress

Practice this when you are not stressed until it becomes a habit – then use it whenever you are getting stressed.

Other Ways to Deal With Stress

- Yoga and other ways to exercise – see the chapters on these in this book
- Learn how to change your life style to eliminate or manage stress, either by yourself using one of the many courses or books available, or by working with a life coach

VII

Conclusions

"It isn't true that you live only once. You only die once. You live lots of times, if you know how."

Bobby Darin

23

Conclusion

My aim in writing this book was to give you the information you need to start taking care of your spinal health.

As we have seen it is a complex subject because the human body is extremely complex. Every client I have seen over the years has had different needs. Each person has been like a complex detective story which has plot twists and turns. In every case the hero is the body itself, with its' amazing ability to work towards perfect health when it is given the right ingredients.

The right ingredients always include:

- A healthy spine and nervous system so that the brain has a clear picture of where the problem are
- The right nutrients so that the body has the building blocks for repair
- Reduced physical, chemical and mental stress so that the body can focus its' energy on repair
- A belief that your body can get better

In this book I have attempted to show you the best ways to put these ingredients in place and I hope you will be able to use this information to improve your health.

If there are any questions I haven't answered please email me at peter@yourspinalhealth.com. I will answer your questions if I can and incorporate your questions and feedback into the next edition of this book so, like the human body, it can constantly improve.

I would also love to hear your success story about how you used this information to transform your health. Again, please email me at peter@yourspinalhealth.com.

Yours in Health

Peter Bennett

24

Frequently Asked Questions

Why do I have to be adjusted so frequently?

Everyone is unique so everyone will have a different care plan set out for them. There are a number of reasons why people need different care

As you have accumulated problems with the nervous system and the spine over years there'll be layers of scar tissue. The scar tissue and tissue damage makes the spine unstable and it tends to revert back to what it is used to. Until the tissues have regrown in the correct place the adjustments have to be frequently repeated to keep the nerves clear.

As you have adapted to your spinal problems over the years you would have developed postural habits - for example holding your head to one side or hitching your pelvis up on one side. Your central nervous system has recorded these postural habits and you have a tendency to revert back to what you think is normal. Again repeated adjustments retrain the postural habits.

Many of the stresses that caused the subluxations in the first place are still ongoing - physical and emotional and chemical. Over time we try to eliminate the stresses but not all of them can be eliminated. Initially we are trying to remove subluxations faster than you can put them back in again.

Do I have to follow the schedule of visits that my spinal health therapist has recommended?

You don't have to do anything you don't want to! The whole approach of spinal health care is to make you the centre of all that we do – you are in control. This also means that you are responsible for your healthcare. Your spinal health therapist will tell you what, in their opinion is the minimal amount of care that you will need to reach your health objectives. If you decide you don't want that level of health just discuss this with your spinal health therapist. However, don't expect to get Rolls Royce health if you are only paying for moped health!

What reactions am I likely to get?

Feeling worse before you get better

Once your innate intelligence is able to start working on the damage to your body your body's response is to break down scar tissue and replace it. The process by which this is done is inflammation. Sometimes inflammation causes pain and you can feel worse before you get better. Sometimes it takes several weeks of care before the nervous system is clear enough for your innate intelligence to break down scar tissue. In these cases clients will initially feel better for a few weeks and then have a few days of pain while the inflammation process proceeds.

Body chemistry changes

As the innate intelligence is dealing with the new information flowing through the nervous system the activity of all the cells in the body can be corrected. This involves changes to body chemistry which can lead to reactions such as emotional changes, heavy sleep or light sleep and changes in the need for medication such as blood pressure medication. The body will always settle itself quickly to as near normal as it can manage so all of these reactions settle down. In some cases the need for medication use will be reduced. Changes in medication should be discussed with your medical doctor.

Retracing of old trauma

I have seen cases where the client has experienced severe physical or emotional trauma at some point in the past. In some cases this trauma has been recorded in the body and will come out and be processed under spinal health care care. Again this is a temporary effect.

The body can change in many ways. Always ask your spinal health therapist about any symptoms or reactions that you are concerned about.

What is that popping noise I sometimes hear during an adjustment?

If a joint has been under stress and been twisted or compressed there will sometimes be a "pop" or "crack" when it releases. As the joint space is opened up the reduction in pressure in the joint fluid causes a gas bubble to form. When the joint settles into it's new position the bubble pops – making the noise. No damage is being caused.

Why does have my spinal health therapist seem to do less work on me in some visits than in others?

The aim of the visit is make sure that any problems in your spine and nervous system are resolved. Ideally we will have got the timing of your appointments about right so you won't have accumulated many problems and there won't be a lot to adjust. On other visits there may be a lot of adjustments because you have been under stress. Remember that we will check everything in your nervous system at every visit.

Why are the appointments short?

Remember that the aim of the visit is make sure that any problems in your nervous system and spine are resolved. The techniques we use have been developed over the last 20 years to quickly identify the issues that your body wants to deal with. When the primary problem is dealt with the secondary problems will often be resolved at the same time. The core part of each visit will often take about five minutes. We allow time for double checking and for you to ask questions and so on, but even so we have found about five to ten minutes is enough time.

The only thing you can't get more of is time. We find that people usually prefer short appointments. It allows them to fit the appointments into their busy lives. It also allows us to be very flexible in moving appointments about to suit you.

However we don't want you to feel rushed. If you feel you need more time with us please ask. We can easily do this and there is no extra charge.

What sort of things can we not help?

There are many causes of health problems other than those related to the spine and nervous system. There may a genetic predisposition to a disease (though keeping stresses out of the body can reduce the severity of the disease). There can also be issues such as strokes or heart disease.

In all situations we are helping your body to be as well as possible. For example if you have had a stroke you will have damaged areas of your brain. We would not be able to do anything about the brain damage. However your body would compensate for the effects of the stroke and cause other symptoms in that way. We would be able to help your body repair the compensation effects – so we would expect you to improve, but we would not expect you to return to the health you had before your stroke.

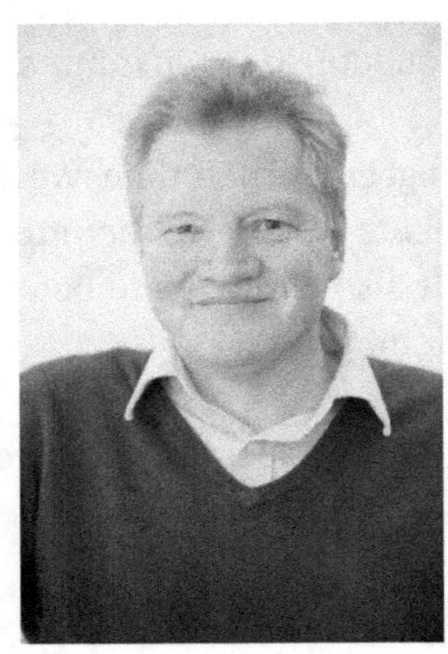

About the Author

Peter Bennett is a chiropractor, life coach, author and speaker. His first degree was in Molecular Biology. After a career in research at The London School of Hygiene and Tropical Medicine and in the pharmaceutical industry he enrolled in the McTimoney Chiropractic College, graduating in 1998.

Over 20 years in practice he developed a holistic system of using the body's responses to find and correct spinal problems and allow the body to heal itself. He teaches this therapy (the Neuro Spinal Reflex Technique) to other therapists.

Peter is married to Janet and they have seven children and live in the beautiful Eden Valley in Cumbria